Top Tips
from the
Baby Whisperer:
Breastfeeding

Top Tips from the Baby Whisperer: Breastfeeding

Tracy Hogg
with Melinda Blau

Vermilion
LONDON

1 3 5 7 9 10 8 6 4 2

Published in 2010 by Vermilion, an imprint of Ebury Publishing

Ebury Publishing is a Random House Group company

The Random House Group Limited Reg. No. 954009

Addresses for companies within the Random House Group can be found at
www.rbooks.co.uk

A CIP catalogue record for this book is available from the British Library

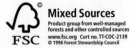

Mixed Sources
Product group from well-managed
forests and other controlled sources
www.fsc.org Cert no. TT-COC-2139
© 1996 Forest Stewardship Council

The Random House Group Limited supports The Forest Stewardship
Council (FSC), the leading international forest certification organisation.
All our titles that are printed on Greenpeace approved FSC certified paper
carry the FSC logo. Our paper procurement policy can be found at
www.rbooks.co.uk/environment

Printed in the UK by CPI Mackays, Chatham, ME5 8TD

ISBN 9780091929732

Text previously published in *The Baby Whisperer Solves All Your Problems*

Copies are available at special rates for bulk orders. Contact the sales development
team on 020 7840 8487 for more information.

To buy books by your favourite authors and register for offers, visit
www.rbooks.co.uk

Contents

Introduction

I have always been proud of my ability to help parents understand and care for their young children, and feel honoured whenever a family asks me into its life. During this time, on my website and in my email inbox, I've been inundated with requests for help: maybe a parent is confused about why their child isn't doing what other children are doing; or maybe they're faced with a deeply entrenched feeding difficulty. Of course, every young child and every family is slightly different. When parents come to me with a particular challenge, I always ask at least one, if not a string of questions, both about the child and about what parents have done so far in response to their situation. Then I can come up with a proper plan of action. In this book, then, I want to show you how to empower yourself as a parent. My goal is to help you understand my thought process and get you in the habit of asking questions for yourself.

Tuning In

Baby whispering begins by observing, respecting and communicating with your baby. It means that you see your child for who she *really* is – her personality and her particular quirks (we all have them) – and you tailor your parenting strategies accordingly.

How often have I witnessed a scene like this: a mother says to her little boy, 'Now Billy, you don't want Adam's truck.' Poor little Billy doesn't talk yet, but if he did I'd bet he'd say, 'Sure I do, Mum. Why else do you think I grabbed it away from Adam in the first place?' But Mum doesn't listen to him. She either takes the truck out of Billy's hand or tries to coax him into relinquishing it willingly. At that point I can almost count the seconds until meltdown!

Don't get me wrong, I'm not saying that just because Billy wants the truck he should be allowed to bully Adam – far from it. What I am saying is that we need to listen to our children, *even when they say things we don't want to hear.*

Those same skills – observing body language, listening to cries, slowing down so that you can really figure out what's going on – are just as important as your baby grows into a toddler and beyond. Those of you who know me undoubtedly recall my love of acronyms, such as E.A.S.Y. (**E**at, **A**ctivity, **S**leep, and time for **Y**ou).

I don't think that coining a series of expressions or acronyms makes child-rearing a snap. I know first-hand that parenting is anything but 'E.A.S.Y.' But in the midst of a tussle with your child or children, it's easy to forget good advice and lapse into old patterns. So I'm trying to give you tools to use when you might not have your wits about you. And here's another acronym for your parental bag of tricks.

Be a 'P.C.' Parent

A P.C. parent is *patient* and *conscious*, two qualities that will serve you well no matter how old your child is. And it's not just problems that require P.C. parenting; so do everyday interactions.

Patience. Today's Big Problem becomes a distant memory a month from now, but we tend to forget that when we're living through it. It takes patience to parent well – those who, in the heat of the moment, take what seems like an easier road, only find out later that it leads them to 'accidental parenting' and a dangerous dead end.

Having a child can be messy and disorderly, too. Therefore, you also need patience (and internal fortitude) to tolerate at least the clutter, spills and finger marks. What toddler manages to drink from a real cup without first spilling pints of liquid on to the floor? Eventually, only a drizzle slips out the side of his mouth and then finally he gets most of it down, but it doesn't happen overnight or without setbacks along the way.

Consciousness. Consciousness of who your child is should begin the moment she takes her first breath outside the womb. Always be aware of your child's perspective. I mean this both figuratively and literally. Squat down and see what the world looks like from her vantage point. Take a whiff of the air. Listen. How loud is the din of the crowd? It's good to expose children to new sights, sounds and people. But, if your infant repeatedly cries in unfamiliar settings, as a conscious parent you'll know that she's telling you: 'Try this with me in another month.'

Consciousness means paying attention to the things you say and what you do with and to your child – and being consistent. So if one day you say, 'No eating in the living room,' and the next night you ignore your son as he does just that, your words will eventually mean nothing.

Finally, consciousness is just that: being awake and being there for your child. Crying is the first language children speak. By turning our backs on them, we're saying, 'You don't matter.' We are their best teachers, and for the first three years, their only teachers. We owe it to them to be P.C. parents – so that they can develop the best in themselves.

But Why Doesn't It Work?

'Why doesn't it work?' is by far one of the most common questions parents ask. Whether a mum is trying to get her seven-month-old to eat solid food or her toddler to stop hitting other kids, I often hear the old 'yes, but' response: 'Yes, I know you told me it will take time, but . . .', 'Yes, I know you said I have to take him out of the room when he begins to get aggressive, but . . .'

Granted, I know that some babies (and some periods of development) are more challenging than others but my baby-whispering techniques *do* work; I've used them myself with thousands of babies. When problems persist, it's usually because of something the parents have done, so you need to ask yourself if one of the following statements applies to you:

You're following your child, rather than establishing a routine. I'm a firm believer in a structured routine (see Chapter 1). You start, ideally, from the day you bring your little bundle home from the hospital. Of course, you can also introduce a routine later, but the older the baby, the more trouble parents often have.

You've been doing accidental parenting. Unfortunately, in the heat of the moment parents sometimes do *anything* to make their baby stop crying or to get a toddler to calm down. Often, the 'anything' – walking, rocking, jiggling or feeding them their favourite 'bad-for-them' treat – turns into a bad habit that they later have to break. And that's accidental parenting.

You're not reading your child's cues. 'He used to be on schedule, and now he's not. How do I get him back on track?' When I hear any version of that phrase, used to be and now is not, it usually means they're paying more attention to the clock (or their own needs) than the baby himself.

You're not factoring in that young children change constantly. I also hear the 'used to be' phrase when parents don't realise that it's time to make a shift; the only constant in the job of parenting is change.

You're looking for an easy fix. The older a child is, the harder it is to break a bad habit caused by accidental parenting, such as demanding a feed, or refusing to sit in a high chair for a proper meal. Be patient.

You're not really committed to change. If you're trying to solve a problem, you have to want it solved – and have the determination and stamina to see it through to the end. If you stick with it, your child will get used to the new way.

Parents sometimes delude themselves. They will insist that they've been trying a particular technique for two weeks and say that it's not working. Often they've tried for three or four days, and it worked, but a few days later they didn't follow through with the original plan. The poor child is then confused.

If you're not going to see something through, don't do it. If you can't do it on your own, enlist backup people.

You're trying something that doesn't work for your family or your personality. If you're not comfortable doing a particular technique, either don't do it, or find ways to bolster yourself, by having the stronger parent take over for a bit or enlisting a relative or a good friend to help.

It ain't broke – and you don't really need to fix it. Babies are individuals. Your child may be eating less than another child the same age or have a smaller-than-average build. If it isn't a concern to your paediatrician, just observe your child.

You have unrealistic expectations. Toddlers can't be managed with the same efficiency you apply to projects at work. Children require care, constant vigilance, and lots of loving time.

Where We Go from Here

I'm not a big fan of age charts and never have been. Children's challenges can't be sorted into neat piles. Still, I have broken down my advice and tailored various techniques according to age groupings to give you a better understanding of how your child thinks and sees the world. You'll notice that the age spans are quite broad. That's to allow for variations among children. In Chapter 1, which deals with E.A.S.Y., I cover only the first five months but this is fundamental to everything that follows. I urge you to read all the stages, because earlier problems can persist and, particularly as children move into toddlerhood, you've got to plan ahead.

You can read this book cover to cover, or just look up the problems you're concerned about and go from there. However, I strongly recommend that you at least read through Chapter 1, which reviews my basic philosophy of a structured routine for your child. Throughout, I've tried to zero in on the most common concerns that parents have when it comes to their child and feeding, and then share with you the kinds of questions I typically ask to find out what's really going on (when I've reprinted emails and website postings, names and identifying details have been changed) and what I would suggest to deal with these concerns. You might be surprised by some of these, but I have lots of examples to demonstrate how successfully they've been applied in other families. So why not at least try them with yours?

CHAPTER ONE

E.A.S.Y. Isn't Necessarily Easy (But It Works!)

Getting Your Baby on a Structured Routine

The Gift of E.A.S.Y.

You probably have a routine in the morning. You get up at roughly the same time, maybe you shower first or have your coffee, or perhaps you take your dog out for a brisk walk. Whatever you do, it's probably pretty much the same every morning. If by chance something interrupts that routine, it can throw off your whole day. Human beings thrive when they know how and when their needs are going to be met and what's coming next.

Well, so do babies and young children. When a new mum brings her baby home from the hospital, I suggest a structured routine straightaway. I call it 'E.A.S.Y.', an acronym that stands for a predictable sequence of events that pretty much mirrors how adults live their lives, albeit in shorter chunks: **E**at, have some **A**ctivity (so the little one doesn't associate eating with sleeping) and go to **S**leep, which leaves a bit of time for **Y**ou. It is *not* a schedule, because you cannot fit a baby into a clock; it's a routine that gives the day structure and makes family life consistent.

With E.A.S.Y., you don't follow the baby; you observe him carefully, tune in to his cues, but you take the lead, gently encouraging him to follow what you know will make him thrive.

Eating affects sleep and activity; activity affects eating and sleeping; sleep affects activity and eating – changes in one usually affect the other two. The acronym simply helps parents remember the order of the routine and, although your baby will transform over the coming months, the order in which each letter occurs does not:

Eat. Your baby's day starts with a feed, which goes from all-liquid to liquids and solids at six months. You're less likely to overfeed or underfeed a baby who's on a routine.

Activity. Infants entertain themselves by staring at the wallpaper. But as your baby develops she will interact more with her environment and move about. A structured routine helps prevent babies from becoming overstimulated.

Sleep. Sleep helps your baby grow. And good naps during the day will make her go for longer stretches at night, because one needs to be relaxed in order to sleep well.

Your time. If every day is different and unpredictable, your baby will be miserable – and you'll barely have a moment for yourself.

Write It Down!

Parents who actually chart their baby's day *by writing everything down* have less trouble sticking to a routine or establishing it for the first time. They see patterns more readily – and will find it clearer to see how sleep and eating and activity are interrelated.

E.A.S.Y. isn't necessarily easy. Some babies adapt more rapidly and readily than others because of their basic temperament, and some special birth conditions (like prematurity or jaundice) or a particular infant's weight mean that E.A.S.Y.

needs to be adapted. Also, some parents misunderstand how to apply E.A.S.Y. For instance, they take 'every three hours' literally and wonder what kind of activity should be done after a feed in the middle of the night. (None – you send him right back to sleep.)

A *structured routine* is not the same thing as a schedule. A schedule is about time slots whereas E.A.S.Y. is about keeping up the same daily pattern – eating, activity and sleeping – and repeating that pattern every day. If you're busy watching the clock, instead of your baby, you'll miss important signals. The most important aspect of E.A.S.Y. is to read your child's signs – of hunger, of fatigue, of overstimulation – which is more important than any time slot. So if one day he's hungry a little earlier or seems to want to eat less than the day before, don't let the clock threaten you. Let your common sense take over.

Guidelines to Get You Started

The E.A.S.Y. Log

When parents come home from the hospital and start E.A.S.Y., I usually suggest that they keep a log (there's one you can download from my website), so that they keep track of exactly what their baby is eating and doing, how long she's sleeping, and also what the mum is doing for herself.

Guidelines for Different Ages

Establishing a routine for the first time gets a bit harder as the baby grows, especially if you've never had structure. So, no matter how old your baby is, it's a good idea to read through all the sections, because, as I will remind you repeatedly, *you can't base strategies solely on age.*

The first six weeks: adjustment time

The first six weeks is the ideal time to start E.A.S.Y., which generally starts out as a three-hour plan. Your baby eats, plays after his feeds, you then set the scene for good napping. You rest while he rests, and when he wakes up, the cycle starts again.

The average baby cries somewhere between one and five hours out of 24 and we should never ignore a baby's cries or, in my opinion, let him cry it out! Instead, we always have to try to figure out what he's telling us. It's understandable, but when the parents of young infants have problems with E.A.S.Y., it's usually because they're misreading their baby's cries, confusing a hungry cry with an overtired cry, for example.

The crying questions
When a six-week or younger baby cries, it's always easier to determine what she wants if you know where she is in her day. Ask yourself:

Is it time for a feed? (hunger)

Is her nappy wet or soiled? (discomfort or cold)

Has she been sitting in the same place or position without a change of scene? (boredom)

Has she been up for more than 30 minutes? (overtired)

Has she had lots of company or has there been a lot of activity in your household? (overstimulated)

Is she grimacing and pulling her legs up? (wind)

Is she crying inconsolably during or as much as an hour after feeds? (reflux)

Is she spitting up? (reflux)

Is her room too hot or cold, or is she under- or overdressed? (body temperature)

Crying often peaks at six weeks, by which time observant parents know what a hungry cry sounds like – a slight cough-like noise in the back of the throat, short to begin with and then as a more steady waa, waa, waa rhythm – compared to an overtired cry, which begins with three short wails, followed by a hard cry, then two short breaths and a longer, even louder cry. They also know their particular baby: while some infants only fuss slightly and 'root' or curl the sides of their tongue, others become absolutely frantic with the first hunger pang. If you put your baby on E.A.S.Y., I guarantee you'll learn her cues more quickly and be better able to determine why she's crying.

	A Typical E.A.S.Y. Day for a 4-Week-Old	
E	7.00	Feed.
A	7.45	Nappy change; some playing and talking; watch cues for sleepiness.
S	8.15	Swaddle and lay your baby in the cot. It may take him 15–20 minutes to fall asleep for his 1st morning nap.
Y	8.30	You nap when he naps.
E	10.00	Feed.
A	10.45	See 7.45 above.
S	11.15	2nd morning nap.
Y	11.30	You nap or at least relax.

A Typical E.A.S.Y. Day for a 4-Week-Old (cont'd)

E	1.00	Feed.
A	1.45	See 7.45 above.
S	2.15	Afternoon nap.
Y	2.30	You nap or at least relax.
E	4.00	Feed.
A	4.45	See 7.45 above.
S	5.15	Catnap for 40–50 minutes to give him enough rest to handle his bath.
Y	5.30	Do something nice for yourself.
E	6.00	1st cluster feed (increasing your baby's intake in the early evening to help his sleep).
A	7.00	Bath, into night clothes, lullaby or other bedtime ritual.
S	7.30	Another catnap.
Y	7.30	You eat dinner.
E	8.00	2nd cluster feed.
A		None.
S		Put him right back to bed.
Y		Enjoy your short evening!
E	10–11	Dream feed (literally feeding your baby in his sleep; at the end of the dream feed, your baby will be so relaxed you can put him down without burping) and cross your fingers until morning!

Note: Whether a baby is breast or bottle-fed, I advise the above routine – allowing for variations in times – until four months old. The 'A' time will be shorter for younger babies and get progressively longer for older ones. I also recommend turning the two 'cluster feeds' into one (at around 5.30 or 6) by eight weeks. Continue the dream feed until seven months – unless he's a great sleeper and makes it through on his own.

Common complaints and probable causes

Complaint: I can't get my baby to conform to a three-hour routine. I can't get her to do even 20 minutes of activity time.

Cause: If your baby weighs less than 3 kg (6½ pounds) at birth, she may need to eat every two hours at first (see E.A.S.Y. by Weight, page 21). Don't try to keep her awake for activities.

Complaint: My baby often falls asleep during feeds and seems hungry an hour later.

Cause: This is common to premature, jaundiced, low birthweight and some simply sleepy babies. You might have to feed more often and definitely have to work at keeping him awake for his feeds. If breastfed, the cause could be poor latch-on, or mum's milk supply (see page 48).

Complaint: My baby wants to eat every two hours.
Cause: If your baby weighs 3 kg (6½ pounds) or more, he may not be eating efficiently. Watch out that he doesn't turn into a 'snacker' (see page 44). If breastfed, the cause could be poor latch-on, or mum's milk supply (see page 48).

Complaint: My baby is rooting all the time and I keep thinking he's hungry, but he only takes a little bit at each feed.
Cause: Your baby may not be getting enough suckling time, so he's using the bottle or breast as a pacifier. He may be turning into a 'snacker' (see page 44). Check your milk supply by doing a yield (see page 52).

Complaint: My baby doesn't take regular naps.
Cause: He may be overstimulated by too much activity. Or you are not persevering with swaddling him and laying him down awake.

Complaint: My baby is a great napper, but she's up frequently at night.

Cause: Your baby has switched night for day and her daytime sleep is robbing her night-time sleep.

Complaint: I never know what my baby wants when he's crying.

Cause: Your baby may have a touchy or grumpy temperament or have a physical problem, such as wind, reflux or colic. Whatever the cause, you and he will do better if he's on E.A.S.Y.

E.A.S.Y. by Weight

E.A.S.Y. was designed for an average-weight newborn – 3–3.5 kg (6½ to 8 pounds) – babies who generally can last three hours between feeds. If your baby weighs more or less, you will have to adjust. This chart shows how birthweight affects your baby's routine. (After four months, even most low-weight babies can last four hours between feeds.) Note the time your baby usually wakes up, and write down approximate times based on your baby's weight and the information in the 'how often' column. Allow for variation – it's not the time slot that matters as much as predictability and order. To simplify, I've left out the 'Y' – time for **Y**ou.

Weight	2.25–3 kg (5–6½ pounds)		3–3.5 kg (6½–8 pounds)		Over 3.5 kg (8 pounds)	
	How long	**How often**	**How long**	**How often**	**How long**	**How often**
Eat	30–40 minutes	Routine repeats every 2 hours during the day, until baby weighs 3 kg (6½ lb), at which point you can switch to an every-3-hour plan. At first these babies can only go 4 hours at night without eating.	25–40 minutes	Routine repeats every 2½–3 hours (for babies on the lower end of average) during the day; 4- to 5-hour stretches at night in the first 6 weeks, by which time you should be working at cutting out the 1 or 2am feed.	25–35 minutes	Routine repeats every 3 hours during the day. By 6 weeks, these babies can generally cut out the 1 or 2am feed and will do a 5- or 6-hour stretch from 11 to 4 or 5am.
Activity	5–10 minutes at first; 20 minutes at 3 kg (6½ lb), gradually extend time to 45 minutes when they are around 3.25 kg (7 lb).		20–45 minutes (includes nappy changing, dressing and, once a day, a bath).		20–45 minutes (includes nappy changing, dressing and, once a day, a bath).	
Sleep	1¼–1½ hours		1½–2 hours		1½–2 hours	

Six weeks to four months: unexpected wake-ups

Compared to the first six weeks at home – the classic post-partum period – during the next two and a half months or so, everyone starts to be on a more even keel.

Common complaints and probable causes

Complaint: I can't get my baby to sleep more than three or four hours during the night.

Cause: She may not be getting enough food during the day, and you also might need to 'tank her up' before bedtime.

Complaint: My baby was sleeping for five or six hours during the night, but now she's waking up more frequently, but always at different times.

Cause: Your baby is probably having a growth spurt and needs more food during the day.

Complaint: I can't get my baby to nap for more than ½ hour or 45 minutes.

Cause: You're probably either not getting him to bed when he first shows signs of fatigue, or you're going in too soon when he first stirs, which doesn't give him a chance to go back to sleep on his own.

Complaint: My baby wakes up at the same hour every night but never takes more than a few ml/ounces when I try to feed him.

Cause: Habitual waking is almost never about hunger. Your baby is probably waking out of habit.

The problem that usually presents in babies this age is a sudden, inexplicable (to the parents, at least) departure from the 'S' part of their routine. Some night waking is naturally due to hunger – babies wake up when their tummies are empty – but that's not always the case. Depending on what the parents do in response to their baby's night waking and nap problems, their well-intentioned actions can sew the seeds of accidental parenting. Say your baby awoke one night and you calmed her by giving her your breast or a bottle – you're inadvertently teaching her that she needs to suckle in order to get back to sleep. Believe me, when she is six months old, you're going to regret that quick fix.

Four to six months: '4/4' and the beginnings of
accidental parenting

At this stage, your baby can hold up her head easily and is
beginning to grasp at things. She is learning to, or already can,
roll over. She can sit up fairly straight with your help, so her
perspective is changing, too. She's more aware of patterns and
routine. She has grown increasingly better at distinguishing
where sounds come from and figuring out cause and effect; she
has a better memory, too.

Because of these strides in development, your baby's daily
routine naturally has to change, too – hence, my '4/4' rule of
thumb, which stands for 'four months/four-hour E.A.S.Y.'.
Most babies are ready at this point to switch from a three- to
four-hour routine.

You can cut one feed because she's taking in more at each
feed, consolidate three naps into two naps (keeping the late
afternoon catnap in either case), and thereby extend your
baby's waking hours. Your baby is probably a more efficient
eater, too, so draining a bottle or breast may take only around
20 to 30 minutes. Including a nappy change, then, the E is 45
minutes at most, but the A is different: now she can stay up a
lot longer.

Comparing the three-hour and four-hour routines

3-hour E.A.S.Y.	4-hour E.A.S.Y.
E: 7.00 Wake up and feed	E: 7.00 Wake up and feed
A: 7.30 or 7.45 (depending on how long feed takes)	A: 7.30
S: 8.30 (1½ hour nap)	S: 9.00 (1½–2 hour nap)
Y: Your choice	Y: Your choice
E: 10.00	E: 11.00
A: 10.30 or 10.45	A: 11.30
S: 11.30 (1½ hour nap)	S: 1.00 (1½–2 hours)
Y: Your choice	Y: Your choice
E: 1.00	E: 3.00
A: 1.30 or 1.45	A: 3.30
S: 2.30 (1½ hour nap)	S: 5.00 or 6.00 or somewhere in between: Catnap
Y: Your choice	Y: Your choice
E: 4.00 feed	E: 7.00 (cluster feed at 7.00 and 9.00, only if going through a growth spurt)
S: 5.00 or 6.00 or somewhere in between: Catnap (approximately 40 minutes) to get Baby through the next feed and bath	A: Bath
	S: 7.30 Bedtime
	Y: The evening is yours!

E: 7.00 (cluster feed at 7.00 and 9.00 if going through a growth spurt)	E: 11.00 Dream feed (until 7 or 8 months, or whenever solid food is firmly established)
A: Bath	
S: 7.30 Bedtime	
Y: The evening is yours!	
E: 10.00 or 11.00 Dream feed	

Your baby won't necessarily conform exactly to these times. Your child might even veer from her own schedule 15 minutes here and there. One day she'll have a shorter nap in the morning and a longer one in the afternoon, or she'll alternate between the two. The important consideration is that you stick to the eat/activity/sleep pattern (now at four-hour intervals).

Common complaints and probable causes

Complaint: My baby finishes her feeds so quickly, I'm afraid she's not getting enough to eat. It also throws off her routine.

Cause: The E may not be a problem at all – some babies are quite efficient eaters by now. You may be trying to keep your child on an E.A.S.Y. plan meant for a younger child – every three hours instead of four.

Complaint: My baby never eats or sleeps at the same time.

Cause: Some variation in your daily routine is normal. But if he's snacking and catnapping – both the result of accidental parenting – he's never getting a good meal or a good sleep. He needs to be on a structured routine suitable for a four-month-old.

Complaint: My baby is still waking up frequently every night, and I never know whether or not to feed him.

Cause: If it's erratic waking, he's hungry and needs more food during the day (see page 69); if it's habitual waking, you have accidentally reinforced a bad habit. You also might have him on a three-instead of four-hour routine.

Complaint: My baby makes it through the night but wakes up at five and wants to play.

Cause: You might be responding too early to his normal early morning sounds and have inadvertently taught him that it's a good idea to wake up so early.

Complaint: I can't get my baby to nap for more than half an hour or 45 minutes – or she refuses to nap at all.

Cause: She may be overstimulated before naptime, or this is the result of a lack of, or improper, routine – or both.

In addition to the above, those seeds of accidental parenting planted earlier now begin to flower in the form of both eating and sleeping problems. Whatever the causes and circumstances, the problem is usually worse at this age because it has been going on longer and, in many cases, because the baby has never been on a routine at all.

Six to nine months: riding out the inconsistencies

We're still looking at a four-hour routine at this stage but, by six months, there's a major growth spurt, too. It's the prime time to introduce solid food, and, by seven months or so, to cut out the dream feed.

Mealtimes are a little longer – and a lot messier – as your baby gets to try a whole new way of eating. Parents have lots of questions and concerns about solid food intake (see Chapter 7). You can't blame them: in the beginning, babies are like eating machines, but at around eight months your baby's metabolism starts to change. She often becomes leaner, losing her baby fat, which has been put on to give her the strength to move around. At this stage it's more important to gauge her diet by quality not quantity.

Now, too, the early evening catnap disappears, and most babies are down to two naps a day. Physical development is key at this stage: by eight months your baby can also hold himself upright, he is becoming more coordinated and he'll be a lot more independent.

The common complaints at this stage are pretty much the same as we saw at four to six months – except, of course, habits are more deeply entrenched and will take a little longer to solve. Otherwise, the biggest issue that crops up at this point is inconsistency. One day she'll eat with gusto, and the next she'd rather skip meals. The key to survival is: if she doesn't stick to a routine, at least you can.

The fact is, because babies nine months and older can stay up for longer stretches without sleeping, it is possible for them to eat, play, eat again, play some more and then go to sleep. In other words, 'E.AS.Y.' becomes 'E.A.E.A.S.Y.'

E.A.S.Y. after Nine Months

Sometime between nine months and a year, your baby will be able to go five hours between feeds. He'll be eating three meals a day, just like everyone else in the family, and have two snacks to tide him over. He can be on the go for two and a half to three hours, and, usually around 18 months – earlier in some children, later in others – get by on one big nap in the afternoon. It's likely he'll be following E.A.E.A.S.Y. at this point, but it's still a structured routine.

Starting E.A.S.Y. at four months or older

If your baby is four months or older, and she's never had a routine, it's time to put her on one. The process is different from that of younger babies for three important reasons:

1. *It's a four-hour routine.* It's important that parents realise they have to adjust the routine to their child's more advanced development (see page 25).

2. *We use my 'pick-up/put-down method' (P.U./P.D.) to make changes.* With babies over four months old, sleep

difficulties are invariably part of the reason why it's impossible to sustain a daily routine. P.U./P.D. can help deal with this (see *The Baby Whisperer Solves All Your Problems*).

3. ***Establishing a structured routine over four months is almost always complicated by accidental parenting.*** Because most parents have already tried other methods, or a medley of methods, the baby has by now got into a bad habit. Therefore, putting an older baby on E.A.S.Y. invariably involves more commitment and work – and consistency.

Making time for change

The thing to keep in mind when introducing a routine for the first time is that there are rarely overnight miracles – three days, a week, even two, but never overnight. When ushering in any new regime to a baby of any age, you're going to get resistance. The first few days will be especially tough because you've already programmed this baby in a different way but, if you're as consistent with the new way as you have been with the old, he'll eventually get used to it.

CHAPTER TWO

Your Baby's Liquid Diet

Feeding Issues in the First Six Months

In the first six months of your baby's life, the 'E' in E.A.S.Y. refers to her liquid diet – breast milk, formula or a combination of the two. We all know that every living creature needs to eat in order to survive. So it's not surprising that eating concerns are second only to sleep when I rifle through the questions put to me by parents. And sleep problems relate to eating issues as well – and vice versa. A well-rested baby eats better; a properly fed baby sleeps better.

If you're one of the lucky ones, your child got off to a good start. Babies are little eating machines at first, they're feeding all the time. Typically, most babies start to take less liquid at around six months as they grow. With growth also comes a change in routine – the 'E' in E.A.S.Y. switches to every four hours during the day (see page 26).

Both breast- and bottle-feeding mums voice similar concerns (especially at the beginning):

Freedom of Choice

The way mothers feed is a matter of choice. Though I support any woman who wants to breastfeed and believe in the benefits of breast milk, I'm an even bigger believer in a mum making a careful, informed – and guilt-free – decision about how to feed rather than trying to do something that makes her unhappy or even frustrated. Some mums can't breastfeed because of diabetes, antidepressant use or other physical reasons. With others, it's a matter of not wanting to. Whatever the reason, that's fine. Formula nowadays has all the nutrients a baby needs.

- How do I know if my baby is getting enough to eat?
- How often do I feed her?
- How can I tell if she's hungry?
- How much is enough?
- If she seems hungry an hour after she's eaten, what does that mean?
- Will I confuse her if I breastfeed and give her a bottle?
- Why does she cry after feeds?
- What's the difference between colic and wind and reflux – and how do I tell whether my baby has any of them?

So now I'll teach you how to figure out what's wrong. Then I'll give you lots of strategies and tips about what to do.

Is My Baby Eating Enough? What's Normal?

When you first bring your baby home, the 'E' in E.A.S.Y. often involves a lot of experimenting, sometimes two steps forward and one step back. The over-riding concern of new mums is, 'Is my baby getting enough to eat? (See the chart Feeding 101 on pages 40–42.) One sure-fire way to find out is to look at weight gain. Check with your doctor what the typical range of weight gain should be, but remember your baby might simply be a small baby (also look for the danger signals – see the box).

With older babies, weight gain can be a tricky matter. If you consult a growth chart, remember that they're designed for *average* children. The old growth charts, originally designed in the fifties, were also based on formula-fed babies, so don't be alarmed if your breastfed baby doesn't measure up (depending on the mother's health and diet, breastfed babies often don't gain as much as formula-fed babies). Also, if your baby starts out less than 2¾ kg

When to Worry About Your Newborn's Weight

Weigh your baby if you're concerned, but not every day. It's normal for a baby to lose up to 10 per cent of her body weight in the first two weeks: she's had a steady flow of food from you through her umbilical cord; now she has to depend on an outside source – you – to feed her. However, you should seek the advice of a paediatrician (and, if you're breastfeeding, a lactation consultant) if your baby:

- loses more than 10 per cent of her birthweight
- doesn't gain her birthweight back within two weeks
- stays at her birthweight for two weeks

(6 pounds), he'll follow a lower-weight curve than a baby who weighs more.

Smaller babies naturally consume less and, in the beginning, have to eat more often (see the E.A.S.Y. by Weight chart on page 22). Babies who are premature or weigh less than 3 kg (6½ pounds) simply don't have the capacity to eat a lot at a feed – their little tummies can't hold enough. They have to eat every two hours. To give yourself a *visual* understanding of this, fill a plastic bag with water to equal the amount of breast milk or formula your baby usually takes, probably 25–50 ml (an ounce or two). Hold the bag next to your baby's tummy. It's easy to see that there's just no room in there to accommodate larger feeds.

Remember that the chart is only a *rough guideline*. On any given day, other factors affect your baby's appetite, such as a poor night's sleep or too much stimulation. Babies are like us: on some days we're hungrier than others, so we eat more; on other days we eat less – if we're tired or just out of sorts. On these 'off' days, your baby will probably eat less, too. On the other hand, if he's in the midst of a growth spurt (see page 67), your baby might eat more.

Also, the ages are approximate: consider this posting from my website; the italicised comments in brackets are mine.

My son, Harry, is six weeks and is 5.1 kg (11 pounds 4 ounces). He has been wanting to eat 175 g (six ounces) of formula every three hours. I have been told that it is way too much. [*By whom, I wonder – her friends, the check-out lady at the supermarket? She doesn't mention her doctor.*] They say the max should be 950 ml (32 ounces), not taking weight into consideration. [*How can you not take a baby's weight into consideration?*] He is maxing out at around 1100–1200 ml (38–40 ounces). We don't know what to do to help Harry interpret his need for food vs. his need to pacify himself.

This is a very smart mum who's listening too much to other people's advice instead of her own inner baby whisperer. She's right to be concerned about not pacifying her son with food, but she needs to tune in to her baby, not her friends. To me, 1100–1200 ml (38–40 ounces) doesn't sound like too much for a big baby. I don't know what he weighed at birth, but I'd guess he's around the 75th percentile, according to universal growth charts. He's only taking around an extra 20 per cent over what someone told her he's 'supposed' to take, and he's got the body to handle it. And it's not like he's snacking (see box, page 44) as he lasts three hours between feeds. He might even start taking 250 ml (8 ounces) as he gets closer to eight weeks. He also might be a baby who needs solid food a little earlier (see page 78).

The bottom line is: look at *your baby*. We always want to look at the individual, not the norm. Books and charts (including the Feeding 101 one) are based on averages, but there are so many exceptions to the rule – babies who eat slower or faster than the norm, babies who eat more or less. By knowing your baby, tuning in to his cues, learning what is developmentally typical, and then using common sense to gauge where your baby stands, you'll probably know what's best. Trust yourself!

Tanking Up

One way of ensuring that your baby eats enough is to increase his intake during the day, before 11pm – 'tanking up'. By doing this, you get more food into his tummy, which, in turn, enables him to sleep through longer stretches at night. Tanking up is also great for growth spurts, those two- or three-day periods when your baby eats more than usual (see pages 67–72).

Tanking up consists of two parts:

1. *Cluster feeding*: at two-hour intervals in the early evening, at 5 and 7 or 6 and 8.

2. *The dream feed*: given somewhere between 10 and 11 (depending on how late you or your partner can stay up). With the dream feed, you literally feed your baby in his sleep. You don't talk to him, or put the lights on. It's easier to do with a bottle, because you just wiggle the nipple into his mouth and that will activate the sucking reflex. It's a little more challenging if you breastfeed. Before you give him your breast, stroke his bottom lip with your little finger or a dummy to get his sucking reflex started. Either way, at the end of the dream feed, your baby will be so relaxed you can put him down without burping.

I recommend tanking up as soon as your baby comes home from the hospital, but you can start using both strategies any time during the first eight weeks and the dream feed until seven or eight months (by which time your baby is drinking between 175 and 250 ml/6 and 8 ounces per feed and getting a fair amount of solid food).

Some infants are harder to tank up than others. They might take early evening feeds but not a dream feed. If that describes your baby, and you have to choose one or the other, *concentrate on the dream feed only.* For example, feed your baby at 6, give her a bath and do the bedtime routine, and top her up at 7 – she'll probably only take a few ml/ounces. Then at 10 or 11 (if you or your partner are normally up that late) try to give her a dream feed – never later than 11. But don't give up after one or two nights; it will take at least three days, and for some infants as long as a week.

Feeding 101

This feeding chart is designed for a baby who weighs 2¾–3 kg (6–6½ pounds) or more at birth. If you're breastfeeding, it also assumes that you haven't had any kind of problems with latch-on or milk supply (see page 48), and that the baby doesn't have any kind of digestive, anatomical or neurological problems. If your baby was premature or underweight, you can still use the chart as a reference, but adjust it. So, for example, if your baby was born a month early, consider him a newborn when he is one month old. Or just go by his weight, not his age.

Age	If bottle-feeding, how much?	If breastfeeding, how long?	How often?	Comments
The 1st 3 days	50 ml (2 ounces) every 2 hours (between 475 and 500 ml/16 and 18 ounces total)	1st day: 5 minutes each breast 2nd day: 10 minutes each breast 3rd day: 15 minutes each breast	All day, whenever baby wants Every 2 hours Every 2½ hours	Breastfeeding mothers need to feed more often to get the milk flowing, which usually happens in the 1st 3 days; on Day 4 switch to single side feeds (see page 49).
Up to 6 weeks	50–150 ml (2–5 ounces) per feed (7 or 8 feeds per day – typical range is 500–725 ml/18–24 ounces total)	Up to 45 minutes	Every 2½–3 hours during the day; cluster feed in the early evening. Your baby should be able to go 4–5 hours during the night, depending on weight and temperament.	At first, bottle-fed babies can go longer between feeds than breastfed babies; it usually evens out at 3–4 weeks, if the mother hasn't had any problems with latch-on or milk supply.
6 weeks–4 months	125–175 ml (4–6 ounces) (6 feeds plus dream feed; typical range is 925–950 ml/24–32 ounces)	Up to 30 minutes	Every 3–3½ hours; by 16 weeks should be able to go 6–8 hours during the night. Don't continue cluster feeding past 8 weeks.	Your goal should be to extend the time between feedings during the day, so that at 4 months, your baby lasts around 4 hours between feeds. But if he's in a growth spurt, and you're breastfeeding, you may need to 'tank up' and/or go back to the 3-hour routine.

Age	If bottle-feeding, how much?	If breastfeeding, how long?	How often?	Comments
4–6 months	150–250 ml (5–8 ounces) per feed (5 feeds plus the dream feed – typical range is 775–1,100 ml/26–38 ounces)	Up to 20 minutes	Every 4 hours; should be able to go 10 hours during the night.	Between 4 and 6 months, some babies' appetite is affected by teething and their newfound mobility, so don't be alarmed if your baby eats less.
6–9 months	5 feeds a day, including solids. Typical range of liquid intake is 950–1450 ml (32–48 ounces). As you introduce solids, liquid consumption declines by the same number of ounces. A baby who once took 1200 ml (40 ounces) of liquid, for example, now takes 425 g (15 ounces) of solids and 750 ml (25 ounces) of liquid. (See page 114 for comparison of solid and liquid food.)	Give food first and then the bottle or 10 minutes on breast. They gulp liquids down quite quickly at this age, so that they can take in more in 10 minutes than they used to in half an hour.	A typical routine: 7.00 Liquid 150–250 ml (5–8 ounces), bottle or breast 8.30 Solids 'breakfast' 11.00 Liquid 12.30 Solids 'lunch' 3.00 Liquid 5.30 Solids 'dinner' 7.30 Breast or bottle before bed	Some babies have early difficulties adapting to solid foods. Your baby may get a runny nose, red cheeks, sore bottom, and possibly diarrhoea, which could indicate a food allergy; check with your paediatrician. Drooling doesn't necessarily mean teething. It starts around 4 months when the saliva glands develop and become mature. When you introduce solids, your baby's liquid intake declines. For every 50 g (2 ounces) of solids, deduct 50 g (2 ounces) of liquid from every feed.

CHAPTER THREE

Troubleshooting: Food-management Issues

The First Six Weeks

Even if your baby is putting on weight, other food issues can develop during the first six weeks. Here are the most common complaints at this stage:

My baby falls asleep during feeds and seems hungry an hour later.
My baby wants to eat every two hours.
My baby is rooting all the time but he only takes a little bit at each feed.
My baby cries during feeds or shortly thereafter.

These are what I call food-management problems, issues that are usually resolved by making sure that your baby is on a structured routine that's appropriate for her birthweight. It's also important for you to learn the difference between hunger cues and other kinds of cries (particularly if your baby has a problem like reflux, wind or colic – see Chapter 4), so

Is Your Baby a Snacker?

Babies can develop a kind of eating pattern in which they never have a good solid meal, but just take in little bits at a time.

How it can happen: The parents confuse the baby's need to suckle with hunger. Instead of giving her a dummy between meals, they give her the breast or a bottle. This starts in the first 6 weeks but can continue for months.

How you know: Your baby is 3 kg (6½ pounds) or more but doesn't last more than 2½–3 hours between feeds, or she never takes more than a few ml/ounces of bottle or 10 minutes of breast at each feed.

that you can get your baby to take full feeds instead of 'snacking' (see box,) and not overfeed her.

What was your baby's birthweight? If your baby was premature or had a low birthweight, he probably needs to feed every two hours. On the other hand, if he weighed over 3 kg (6½ pounds) at birth, and he's not lasting more than two hours between feeds, either he's not getting enough at each feed or he's pacifying instead of eating.

Are you bottle- or breastfeeding? With bottle-feeding, there's less guesswork involved than with breastfeeding, because you can actually see what your baby takes in. If she's 3 kg (6½ pounds) or more and drinks 50–150 ml (2–5 ounces) of formula, but seems hungry an hour after a feed, she probably just needs to suckle – give her a dummy. If she still seems hungry, she might need more at each feed.

If you're breastfeeding, you must gauge how long a feed takes: most infants up to six weeks old will nurse at least 15 or 20 minutes at each feed – any less and they're probably snacking. But also make sure that your baby is latched on properly, and that your milk supply is adequate (see page 48).

How often do you feed your baby? Average-sized and bigger babies need to eat every 2½–3 hours in the beginning, no less, no longer. (See page 38 regarding tanking up.) If your baby 'is hungry every hour', your feeds may be too short (see below) or your baby isn't getting enough to eat at each feed. (It's also possible that your baby is going through a growth spurt (see pages 67–72).) If you're bottle-feeding, the solution is simple: add 25 ml (an ounce) to each of your baby's feeds. If you're breastfeeding, it may be that your baby needs more milk than you're producing or that the baby isn't latched on properly and therefore isn't getting much out of your breast. When babies feed for only 10 minutes at a time, your body will think that you don't need to

Is Your Baby a Snacker? *cont'd*

What to do: If breastfeeding, first check for a proper latch-on and do a yield (see page 52) to rule out those problems. And make sure that you feed from only one side at a time, which ensures that your baby gets to the richer hind milk (see page 49). If your baby starts crying after 2 hours, use a dummy to hold her off – just 10 minutes the first day, 15 the second, so she lasts a bit longer between feeds. By doing this, you'll also increase your milk supply. If this is impossible, just give her a smaller snack – less time on the breast, or 25 ml (1 ounce) less of the bottle; she'll make that up at the next feed. It may take 3 or 4 days, but if you're consistent, she'll become a feeder . . . especially if you catch it in the first 6 weeks.

make as much milk, so over a two- or three-week period your supply will diminish and eventually dry up (see pages 98–99).

How long does a feed usually last? During the first six to eight weeks, an average-weight baby's feedings take 20 to 40 minutes. Although bottle-fed babies can fall asleep on the job, too, once they weigh 3 kg (6½ pounds) or more, they're less likely to pass out during a feed than a breastfed baby. Breastfed babies tend to get sleepy around 10 minutes into a feed because they've had a slug of the 'quencher', the fore part of the milk that is rich in oxytocin, a hormone that acts like a sleeping pill (see the box on page 49).

Falling asleep on the job every now and then is okay but, if the sleepy-baby pattern continues for more than three feeds, you might be turning your baby into a snacker. Also, if a baby learns to associate suckling with sleep, it will be harder to teach him to fall asleep on his own. Try to keep your baby up after a feed, even for as little as five minutes. Change her nappy or just talk to her. Spend only 10 to 15 minutes trying to wake her, by which time the oxytocin should have made its way through her system. After that, consider her into the 'S' part of E.A.S.Y. And try again at the next feed. Be persistent.

What if she was up all night and is tired? Why do you think she was up all night? She was demanding to be fed because she's catching up on the food she wasn't getting during the day. If you let the pattern persist, by the time she's four months old, you'll be wondering if you'll ever get her to sleep through the night.

Between feeds, are you giving your baby suckling time? Babies need suckling time, especially in the first three months. So try a dummy between feeds to stretch the times between them gradually.

Does your baby cry a lot after meals or at least within the hour? Infants who cry during or shortly after feeds *aren't* crying because they're still hungry. First, rule out problems in your own body like a poor milk supply or blocked duct. If that's fine, it probably means your baby is in pain and has wind or oesophageal reflux (baby heartburn) – see Chapter 4.

How long is your baby's activity period? Remember that we're talking about babies six weeks and under. Some infants, especially small ones, can only stay up five or 10 minutes after a feed; if you keep them up too long, they'll become overstimulated. Your baby may not be eating enough to sustain her activity and can't take a meaningful nap because her tummy's empty. You need to extend her feeds and shorten her awake time.

Avoid (or Correct) Poor Latch-on and Low Milk Supply

If you're healthy when you're pregnant, your body gets revved up to produce milk and, when your baby is born, all the mechanisms are in place to feed her what she needs. It's a natural process, but not every woman or baby necessarily takes to it immediately. You're not wrong or bad if you need help.

When new mums come to me with so-called breastfeeding problems during the first six weeks it usually boils down to either a *poor latch-on* in which the baby's mouth is not positioned in a way that allows her to get the most milk, or an *insufficient milk supply*. These two problems can, of course, be related – if your baby isn't latching on properly, your body will begin to produce less milk and you'll have an insufficient milk supply.

As the Feeding 101 chart (pages 40–42) indicates, the first few days are different for breastfed babies, because Mum's breasts first secrete colostrum (see box, page 49) until her milk comes in. To get the maximum benefit of colostrum you feed *all day* on the first day, five minutes on each side. The second day, you feed every two hours, 10 minutes on each side, and the third every two-and-a-half hours, 15 to 20 minutes on each side. When your baby takes in colostrum she has to use a lot of energy to suck it in, which can be especially hard for babies who weigh less than 2¾ kg (6 pounds). But this frequent suckling is critical because, the faster your milk comes in, the less chance you'll get engorged.

Once your milk comes in, do single-side feeding. In other words, don't switch to the other breast until you've emptied the first one. Breast milk has three parts: a watery liquid; a bluish white liquid; and a thick yellowish creamy substance. The watery part – the quencher – comes out during the first 10 minutes of a feed. So, if you switch sides after 10 minutes, you're not only going to put your baby to sleep, you're giving her a double dose of quencher and none of the later, nutritious, creamier parts. In my opinion, babies whose mums switch sides are often the babies who turn into snackers, and they may develop digestive problems too,

If Breast Milk Were Labelled . . .

When you buy formula, it has a label. But breast milk changes as your baby does:

Colostrum: For the first 3 or 4 days, your baby will be nourished by colostrum, a thick, yellowish substance that's like a power bar. In it are all the antibodies your child needs to stay healthy.

Quencher: Once your milk starts to come in, the first 5–10 minutes consists of a watery substance that's high in lactose and slakes your baby's thirst. It's also rich in oxytocin, which acts like a sleeping pill.

Fore milk: The next 5–10 minutes, a high-protein liquid comes through. It's good for bones and brain development.

Hind milk: 15–18 minutes later comes the fat-rich cream of breast milk. High in calories and thick, it helps your baby gain weight.

because the fore milk is rich in lactose, too much of which can cause tummy aches.

Make sure your baby is latching on properly. Buy yourself a box of those little round plasters, each around 12–20 mm (½–¾ inch) in diameter. Place one 25 mm (1 inch) above your nipple, and one 25 mm (1 inch) below. Prop your baby up on a firm pillow or breastfeeding cushion and lay him in the fold of your arm level with your breast, so he doesn't have to strain his neck. Place your thumb on the top target and your forefinger on the bottom one and squeeze. Then, gently take your baby's head and thrust the nipple into his mouth. To make sure that your baby is latched on correctly, watch yourself in the mirror or ask someone else to observe how your baby's lips grasp on to your nipple:

- ✓ Your baby's mouth should be wide and positioned squarely on the nipple.

- ✓ The baby's lips should form a tight flange around the nipple and areola.

- ✓ The baby's bottom lip should not be tucked in.

- ✓ He should be full on your nipple, rather than just on top of it.

- ✓ Your fingers should be on the 'targets' to help the baby get the full nipple into his mouth.

The surest sign of an improper latch-on is in *your* body – sore, even bleeding, nipples. Trust your body's signals. A little soreness in your nipple in the first two or three days is normal, but if discomfort lasts longer or get worse, something probably *is* wrong:

- If it pinches or it hurts when your baby suckles, she isn't latched on correctly.

- If your nipple develops a blister, your hands are in the wrong position.

- If you physically feel sick – fever, chills, night sweats – and have any kind of pain or swelling in your breasts, those are all signs of problems, such as engorgement or a blocked duct (which could lead to mastitis, or inflammation of the mammary gland).

- If you have a fever or are otherwise symptomatic longer than a week, seek the help of a doctor. You could also seek help from a health visitor or lactation consultant.

If your baby weighed less than 2¾ kg (6 pounds) at birth, feed more frequently, even after the first four days. Milk-supply problems are common with small infants, because your body is

How to Increase Your Milk Supply

The key is to stimulate the sinuses in your breast, either by pump or by your baby's mouth.

No pump method: Put your baby on your breast every 2 hours for a few days, and that will get your milk flowing. The baby stimulates the sinuses, which sends a signal to the brain to produce milk. Your baby will then be able to go 2½–3 hours between feeds, because he's getting the proper amount to eat. (If feeds don't automatically extend within the next 4 days, make sure he's not becoming a snacker (see page 44).)

designed to sustain a 3 kg (6½ pound) or larger baby. When the baby doesn't suck as strongly or take in as much milk, the mum's body reduces her milk supply. The remedy is to feed every two hours to keep the baby's weight up and keep Mum's milk flowing. In extreme cases, such as with premature or very underweight babies, it's best to pump between feeds to keep the baby's milk supply going (see box).

If you're worried about supply, do a yield to find out how much you're producing. Once a day, 15 minutes before a feed, pump your breasts and see how much comes out. Let's say it's 50 ml (two ounces), your baby would probably have got 85 ml (three ounces) (physical suckling is more efficient than any pump). Then give her that breast milk in a bottle, or by a syringe or pipette if you haven't introduced a bottle yet. You could also put your baby on your breast, let him empty the rest, and then give him whatever milk you pumped.

Make sure you get enough sleep and eat well. Breast milk changes as a result of the mother's lifestyle – too little sleep (and diet) can deplete your supply or even reduce the caloric value of your breast milk. Double your intake of liquid – drink 16 glasses of water or an equivalent beverage a day; consume an extra 500 calories, 50 per cent from carbohydrates, 25 to 30 per cent each from fats and proteins – in addition to your daily intake to replenish the energy that your body is using to manufacture breast milk. These are averages; consult your obstetrician or a nutritionist if you're in doubt.

> **How to Increase Your Milk Supply** *cont'd*
>
> *Pumping method:* Pump straight after feeding or wait for an hour after the baby is fed and then pump. It might seem strange but, by pumping, you empty the reservoir completely. At the next feed your baby's suckling will then signal your body to produce more milk. After 3 days your milk supply should increase.

Recently, I got a call from 35-year-old Maria, a new mum who was wondering why her eight-week-old baby, who'd started out on a good solid three-hour routine, was now going back to eating every one-and-a-half hours. As it turned out, the problem was Mum's no-carbohydrate diet, and her two-hour-a-day exercise routine, which, even if she'd had a different diet, was too active for a nursing mum.

Supplement with formula if you have to. Many mums are desperate to breastfeed, but sometimes we *have* to supplement a baby's feeds with formula, at least until our milk supply increases. Pumping will increase supply until you can gradually feed him less formula and more breast milk.

> IMPORTANT REMINDER: Unless you're going into surgery and you physically won't be around to feed your baby, don't pump more than an extra three days' worth of breast milk. As your baby grows and changes, the content of your breast milk changes, too. Last month's breast milk may not be suitable for this month's baby.

Be wary if feeds regularly take less than 10 or 15 minutes. First, rule out improper latch-on or poor milk supply: **Have you taken a yield to see how much breast milk you're actually producing? Are your nipples sore? Are you getting engorged?** 'Yes' to either the second or third question might indicate that the baby isn't latched on properly. You probably have blocked ducts; contact a midwife or doctor.

But where I've seen a lot of breastfeeding mums go wrong in the first six weeks is that they don't leave the baby on long enough to get a full feed. When, 10 minutes or so into the feed, his eyes start closing, a child's mother assumes that the feed is over and that her little boy is into the 'S' part of the routine. She doesn't realise that he couldn't have got to the fatty hind milk that starts flowing around 15 minutes into a feed. When he wakes again about 10 minutes later, the oxytocin has made its way out of his system, and he barely has enough in his stomach to sustain him. He cries; his mother believes he can't be hungry and tries everything else she can to calm him. After 20 or 30 minutes of crying, any young baby will be so exhausted that he will fall back to sleep. But – and this is what drives Mum crazy – he doesn't *stay* asleep.

Instead, use my wake-up techniques (see page 46) to rouse your child when he nods off during a feed. Your child should begin eating proper meals, gaining weight and, of course, sleeping better as well.

So pay attention to the length of feeds but also remember that all babies are different. Some babies are efficient eaters right from the start. The key is whether she's lasting three hours between feeds – if she is, she's not snacking. Unless her weight is unusually low, she's presumably taking enough food to sustain her.

Baby Whisperer's Best Advice: Breast *and* Bottle

I always tell mums who breastfeed to introduce their baby to a bottle as well. I recommend starting as soon as your baby has latched on correctly, and you've established a good flow, which for most mums is around 2 or 3 weeks. Then give a bottle at least once a day.

Now I know that some mums are advised to breastfeed exclusively, or at least to wait until the baby is 6 months old before giving a bottle – this is because of so-called nipple confusion or because their own milk might dry up. Rubbish! I've never had either of those problems with my babies.

Besides, it isn't just a matter of your baby's health. You also have to factor in your own needs and your lifestyle – think ahead. Look at the critical questions below – if you answer yes to any of them, consider introducing a bottle in the first few weeks. (If you've already missed that window, see pages 98–104.)

Would you like someone else to be able to feed your baby too?

A baby who takes breast and bottle gives Mum a break and can be fed by others, who then also get an opportunity to cuddle, talk to, and bond with the baby.

Are you planning to go back to work before your baby is a year old?

If you're going back to work, and your baby is not used to both breast and bottle, you risk a hunger strike (see pages 101, 102–103).

Are you planning to put your baby in day care before he's a year old?

Most facilities won't take a baby who can't be bottle-fed.

Now that you've started breastfeeding, are you sure you want to continue?

There is no magic date or optimal time to wean a baby. Whenever you decide to quit, it will be a smoother transition if your baby is already used to a bottle.

Do you plan to breastfeed for a year or less?

You *don't* want to start introducing a bottle at 8 or 10 months for the first time. If you do, you're likely to find your baby resistant.

CHAPTER FOUR

Troubleshooting: Gastric Distress

Painful Feeds

The worst thing about any child's gastrointestinal problem is that it sets in motion a series of events and emotions that only make the problem worse and more difficult to deal with: Mum and Dad often feel helpless because they can't figure out the problem; they start questioning their own skills; they in turn become tense, worried and anxious while feeding.

Infants' digestive systems are very immature. When parents tell me that their baby is 'crying all the time', the first thing I suspect is some kind of gastric problem: wind, reflux (baby heartburn) or colic.

Wind, reflux and colic are all different conditions (though the first two are often mistaken for the third). The following should help you understand as much as anyone knows:

The Crying Game

To determine why a baby is in distress, I ask specific questions about crying. (Of course, I also need to ask birthweight, eating patterns, activities, sleeping habits – to rule out hunger, tiredness, overstimulation or, more likely, a combination of the three.)

When does he usually cry?

- If he cries after feeds, it's probably wind or reflux.
- If he cries like clockwork at the same time every day, it could be colic (if the other two conditions have been ruled out).
- If his crying is erratic and random, it might be his temperament – certain types of babies cry more than others.

Wind

WHAT IT IS: Air that your baby swallows during feeding. Some babies like the sensation of swallowing, so they'll gulp air even when they're not eating. When that air gets trapped in the intestine, it causes pain, because there's no way for the body to break it down. Your baby just has to eliminate it by passing wind or burping.

WHAT TO LOOK FOR: Your baby will probably bring his legs up to his chest. He'll scrunch up his face. There will also be a definite pitch and tone to his cry – it's an intermittent crying and he'll look like he's panting – as if he's about to belch. He might also roll his eyes and wear an expression (between cries) that almost looks like a smile.

WHAT TO DO: ***When you burp your baby***, rub upward on his left side (the soft part under his left rib is where his stomach is) using the heel of your palm. If that doesn't work, pick him up with his arms dangling over your shoulder and legs straight down. This gives the air a direct path. Rub upward, as if you're smoothing a piece of wallpaper to get the air bubble out.

Lay your baby on his back. This will help your baby expel the wind; pull up his legs, and do a gentle bicycling motion.

Hold him against you and pat his bottom, which gives him a sense of where to push.

Lay him across your forearm, face down, and put gentle pressure on his tummy with your palm.

Wrap a makeshift cummerbund around his middle by folding a receiving blanket into a 100-mm (four-inch) band and tucking it snugly – but not too tightly – around his middle.

The Crying Game *cont'd*

What does his body look like when he cries?
- If he pulls his feet up to his chest, it's probably wind.
- If he goes rigid and arches his back, it could be reflux, but it also could be his way of shutting out the world.

What comforts him when he cries?
- If burping him or bicycling his legs eases his crying, you probably helped him pass a wind bubble.
- If sitting him upright – say in a car seat or swing – does the trick, it could be reflux.
- Motion, the sound of running water, the vacuum might distract a baby who has colic, but more often there's very little one can do to console a colicky baby.

Reflux

WHAT IT IS: Baby heartburn, sometimes accompanied by vomiting. In extreme cases, there can be complications and the baby can regurgitate blood-tinged liquid. When your baby eats, food goes into the mouth and down the oesophagus. If the digestive system is working properly, the sphincter – the muscle that opens and closes the stomach – allows the food to drop in and keeps it there. With reflux, the sphincter doesn't close properly after opening. The food doesn't stay down and, to make it worse, stomach acid comes up with it, burning your baby's oesophagus.

WHAT TO LOOK FOR: One or two episodes of spitting up should not alarm you. All babies have reflux at one time or another, some have it more often, and some infants are simply more sensitive to digestive issues. I ask: **Was he breach? Did he have the cord wrapped around his neck during delivery? Was he premature? Was he jaundiced? Was he a low-birthweight baby? Did Mum have a C-section? Have any of the adults or other children in the family had reflux?** A yes to any of those questions points to a higher chance of reflux.

If she has reflux, your baby will have trouble getting through her feeds. She might splutter and choke, because her sphincter has stayed shut, making it impossible for her to get food down in the first place. Or, she might spit up or projectile-vomit a few minutes after eating. Sometimes you'll also see a watery cottage-cheese spit-up as long as an hour after a feed.

She might have explosive poos. Like a windy baby, she might also gulp air, but, with reflux, the gulp is accompanied by a little squeaky noise. Reflux babies are often hard to burp. Another key sign is that the only way they feel comfortable is when they're sitting up or are held upright on a shoulder. Attempts to lay them down result in bouts of hysterical crying.

The vicious circle with oesophageal reflux is that, the more tense a baby is and the more crying he does, the more likely it is that he'll have a spasm and that the acid will come up his oesophagus and make him even more uncomfortable. You try every trick in the book and nothing calms him. Chances are you tend to jiggle him up and down to comfort him or pat his back to burp him, but this only helps the acid move up the oesophagus.

You might attribute his crying and his discomfort to colic or wind without realising he has heartburn. You get confused and

It's a Myth

The old-fashioned diagnosis for reflux included constant spitting up and/or projectile vomiting. But we now know that some babies have the pain and the problem without those symptoms. Because of this confusion, reflux can still be misdiagnosed as colic. That might explain why some cases of colic 'magically' disappear at around four months. By then, the immature sphincter muscle starts to strengthen – the more it's used, the stronger it gets – and the baby finds it easier to eat and digest.

abandon your routine because you're having trouble reading his cues. Meanwhile, your baby is exhausted. He gets hungry again from all that crying, so you try to feed him again. And so the cycle continues.

WHAT TO DO: If your paediatrician says it's colic, get a second opinion from a paediatric gastroenterologist, especially if the adults in your family or other children have gastrointestinal problems. Reflux runs in families. Often a health history and thorough examination is enough to diagnose the problem without lab tests. In extreme cases, or if your doctor thinks there might be complications from your child's reflux, various tests may be performed – X-ray with a barium swallow, ultrasound, endoscopy, oesophageal pH study. The specialist will determine if your baby has reflux, gauge its severity, and can usually estimate how long your baby's reflux will last, as well as giving you guidelines to manage it and, commonly, medication: baby antacids and relaxants.

But there are also things you can do besides taking him for rides in the car:

Elevate the cot mattress. Raise it to a 45-degree angle to make the head higher by using a baby wedge or a couple of books. Babies with reflux do best when propped up and swaddled.

Do not pat your baby when burping him. You'll make him vomit or he'll start crying, which starts the vicious circle. Rather, gently rub in a circular motion on the left side of his back. Rub upward with baby's arm straight over your shoulder so there's a clear passage up the oesophagus. If, after three minutes, he doesn't burp, stop burping him. If there's air in there, he'll start being fussy. Gently lift him forwards and the air will probably come out.

Pay attention to feeds. Avoid overfeeding your baby or feeding him too quickly (which is more likely to happen on a bottle). If a bottle-feed takes less than 20 minutes, the hole in the nipple may be too large; switch to a slow-release nipple. If he starts fussing after a feed, use a dummy to calm him rather than feed again, which will only make him more distressed.

Don't rush to give him solid food. In my opinion, if you fill his tummy too much, it will give him even worse heartburn. He'll stop feeding if he has pain.

Try to stay calm yourself. Reflux tends get better at around eight months, when the sphincter is more mature and your baby is eating more solid foods. Most babies outgrow reflux in the first year; the most severe cases can continue through age two, but they're in the minority. Take the steps you can to make him comfortable and accept that your baby isn't going to conform to a normal eating pattern – at least not for now.

Colic

WHAT IT IS: Not even doctors agree about what colic is or how to define it. Most consider it a complex clustering of symptoms characterised by loud, excessive and inconsolable crying, which seems to be accompanied by pain and irritability. Some see it as an umbrella that covers: *digestive problems* (allergies to food, wind or reflux), *neurological problems* (hypersensitivity or highly reactive temperament) and *unfavourable environmental conditions* (nervous or neglectful parents, tension in the home).

Babies diagnosed with colic can have any – or all – of these conditions, but not all will necessarily have true colic. Some paediatricians still use the old 3/3/3 rule: three non-stop hours of crying, three days a week, for three consecutive weeks, which statistically adds up to about 20 per cent of all babies. First-born infants seem to be affected with colic more often than later children. It usually begins within 10 days to three weeks after birth, and lasts until three or four months of age, at which time it generally disappears on its own. Some studies now suggest that colic has nothing to do with stomach pain at all; instead, it's caused by a baby's inability to console himself when dealing with all the things that bombard his senses.

WHAT TO LOOK FOR: When a mother suspects that her baby is 'colicky', I first rule out wind and reflux. Even if they are considered subsets of colic, at least you can take steps to alleviate them. Despite their crying, colicky babies put on weight, whereas many babies with reflux lose weight. Babies with reflux will tend to arch backwards during a crying spell; with wind, he pulls his legs up. With both reflux and wind, spells typically occur within an hour or less of the last feed, whereas colic isn't necessarily related to feeds. Severe bouts of loud crying that last for several hours at a time, often at the same time of day every day and with no apparent reason could suggest colic in your child.

WHAT TO DO: The trouble is, all babies cry. They cry when they're hungry or upset or when you change their routine. Your paediatrician might prescribe a mild sedative (knock-out drops), advise you to avoid overstimulating your baby, or suggest various tricks of the trade like running water, the vacuum or your hair dryer to distract your baby.

Some will also suggest breastfeeding more frequently, which I categorically *don't* recommend because, if the problem is in your baby's gastric system, overfeeding makes it worse.

Whatever the suggestions, remember that true colic has no 'cure'. You pretty much have to ride it out. If you're not equipped to do this, call in the reserves, and take lots of breaks so that you don't get to breaking point yourself.

CHAPTER FIVE

Growth and Eating Changes

Six Weeks to Six Months

Six Weeks to Four Months: Growth Spurts

Many of the early feeding wrinkles are ironed out by this stage. Your baby is probably a bit more consistent, eating and sleeping better – unless of course she's plagued by gastro-intestinal problems or she's very sensitive to her environment. In that case, hopefully you've learned to accept her temperament and are more tuned in to her cues. You also know the best way of feeding her and keeping her comfortable after meals. At this stage, I get variations on the following two complaints:

> *I can't get my baby to sleep more than three or four hours during the night.*
>
> *My baby was sleeping for five or six hours during the night, but now she's waking up more frequently, always at different times.*

Parents think they're calling me about a sleeping issue but, to their surprise, both problems are related to food at this stage. It depends on birthweight and temperament but, by eight weeks, babies should be sleeping at least five hours through the night, if not six. With babies who have already started to sleep longer stretches, night waking is commonly due to a *growth spurt – a period, typically lasting a day or two, when your baby's body demands more food.*

If your baby is average-sized or heavier and has never been able to get to sleep more than three or four hours, I first ask, **How many naps and for how long is your baby sleeping during the day?** But if her naps aren't too long and she still can't put more than three or four hours together at night, it probably means she needs to be eating more food during the day and to have a full tummy when you put her to bed. If you haven't already done so, I would suggest tanking up (see page 38).

Where a baby has been sleeping through for five or six hours and now starts waking at different times, it usually means that she's going through a growth spurt. Growth spurts happen for the first time between six and eight weeks and recur thereafter about once a month or every six weeks. The one at five or six months is usually a signal that it's time to introduce solid food. (Growth spurts can occur earlier in bigger babies, which can be confusing. Use your judgement – he obviously needs more to sustain him.)

Growth spurts in breastfeeding babies shouldn't be confused with improper latch-on or a problem with Mum's milk supply, both of which also cause night-waking but usually happen earlier than six weeks (see page 48). The critical question is: **Does she wake at the same hour every night, or is her waking pattern erratic?** If it's erratic, it's usually a growth spurt:

> I've just started my seven-week-old Olivia on E.A.S.Y., which she has taken to really well. But since we've started, her sleeping schedule at night has become more erratic. Before she would wake up at 2.45. But lately she seems to have no consistency despite her eating and sleeping at relatively the same time during the day. We have kept a log and we can't really find anything that we are doing differently each night that would cause her to sometimes wake up at 1 and other times not until 4.30. Is there anything we can do to promote her to sleep until at least 2.45 like she used to?

In a case like Olivia's, I know it is definitely a growth spurt, because she had been a pretty good eater and sleeper all along, and she's been on a routine. Another real tip-off is that her sleeping schedule at night had become *more erratic*. Because her waking happened to coincide with the parents putting Olivia on E.A.S.Y., they naturally assume her sudden sleep disturbances has something to do with the new routine. But their baby is just hungry.

Let's say instead that we're talking about a baby who's never slept well. She still wakes up twice a night. She, too, might be going through a growth spurt, but she also could be getting into a very bad sleep pattern, and Mum and Dad reinforce it by feeding her when she wakes. So how do you know the difference?

One clue is the waking pattern. But the best clue is food intake: when Mum tries to feed her, if she's having a growth spurt, she will take a full feed because her body needs the extra food. If she doesn't take more than a few ounces, it's pretty conclusive evidence that it's a bad sleeping pattern.

The prescription for a growth spurt is always the same: increase food during the day and, if you haven't already started doing so, add a dream feed at night. With bottle-fed babies, we increase by 25 ml (one ounce) the amount of formula you give during the day. With breastfed babies, it's a little trickier, because you increase the feed *time* rather than the amount. So, if your baby is on a three-hour routine, bump it up a bit to every 2½ hours. With an older baby who's on a '4/4' routine (see page 25), go back to feeding every 3 or 3½ hours. This advice might sound like you're moving backwards but remember that it's just a *temporary* measure. By feeding more often, you will let your body know that it has to manufacture more milk and, in a few days, you will be producing enough milk to satisfy his new needs.

Growth spurts can disrupt your baby's routine at bedtime, during the middle of the night, or when you put them down for a nap. If he isn't fed, a child will start to associate hunger with his bedroom. If you were sent to your room before you finished your dinner, there's a good chance you wouldn't want to go to your room, either!

If your baby is resistant to the dream feed, you also might want to re-evaluate how you're feeding him during the day. One little lad I cared for, Christian, was nine weeks old at the time, and no matter how hard his mum and I tried, he wouldn't take that 11pm feed. For weeks, Mum had been feeding him at 5 and 8 and then trying to feed him again at 11, which was only three hours later. Chris was almost 4 kg (9 pounds) at that point, so he wasn't hungry at 11. But then he woke up at 1am starving.

We decided only to give him 50 ml (2 ounces) at 5pm

Dream Feeding Too Late

Remember that a dream feed should never be later than 11. Otherwise, you're cutting into the night, and a baby will then eat that much less during the day, and he'll get into the habit of waking at night from hunger.

Janet called me because her son was waking up at 4.30 or 5 every morning. The problem was, she was feeding four-month-old Kevin his dream feed between midnight and 1am. At his age and for his size (he was 8 pounds at birth), he should have been sleeping at least five, if not six, hours during the night. But, because Janet was unwittingly disrupting his sleep with a too-late dream feed, he slept fitfully. Then, to make matters worse, Janet fed him when he woke in the small hours of the morning, which only reinforced his waking *habit*. I suggested that she gradually move the dream feed to 10 or 10.30, but stop feeding him when he woke, and to add an ounce to each of his daytime bottles.

instead of the 200 ml (7 ounces) he usually took, and moved the 8pm feed back an hour, to 7pm, and only gave him 175 ml (6 ounces) instead of his usual 250 ml (8 ounces). In other words, we took away 200 ml (7 ounces) altogether from his evening feeds. He had an activity afterwards – his bath – and, by the time he was massaged, swaddled and put to bed, he was pretty tired. Then we took the dream feed to 11, which meant that now there were four hours between his early evening feeds – Chris took a full 250 ml (8 ounces). At that point, we also figured he needed more food during the day, so we upped his feeds 25 ml (1 ounce) per bottle. Thereafter, he lasted through the night from the dream feed to a 6.30am wake-up.

Four to Six Months: A More Grown-up Eater

This is a stage of relative calm in the eating department if you've got your baby on a structured routine. She'll still be crying for her meals, but, depending on her temperament (and how you respond to her), your baby will probably have a less desperate tone. Some babies will even play on their own in the morning, rather than wake their parents with a 'Feed me!' wail. These are often the concerns at this stage:

> *My baby never eats at the same time of day.*
> *My baby finishes her feeds so quickly, I'm afraid she's not getting enough to eat. It also throws her off schedule.*
> *My baby doesn't seem interested in eating any more.*

I'll bet you can guess the first question I ask: **Is your baby on a structured routine?** If the answer is 'no' – and it usually is when parents say their baby never eats at the same time every day – you can't blame eating problems on the baby. And, if your baby is always eating at random, I'll bet he never gets a good sleep either. (See 'Starting E.A.S.Y. at Four Months or Older', pages 31–32.)

If the baby has been on a routine: **How long does your baby go between feeds?** If she's feeding every two hours, it's a snacking problem, because no four-month-old or older baby needs to eat that often. At almost five months old, Maura was still feeding every two hours, even through the night. A friend had suggested putting cereal in Maura's bottle 'to help her get through the night' – an old wives' tale if I ever heard one. As Maura had never had solids, all that did was constipate her, and she still woke up looking for her mum's breast.

Instead, I advised her parents to tank Maura up at 6, 8, 10, and then *not* feed her at night – no matter what. The first night she naturally woke up screaming several times between 10 and 5, but they didn't cave in. Dad used my pick-up/put-down method (see *The Baby Whisperer Solves All Your Problems*) to get Maura back to sleep each time, but it was a hard night, especially for Mum, who thought she was starving her baby. In the morning, though, for the first time in a long time (maybe ever) Maura took a full half-hour feed at 5am. For the rest of the day, Maura ate pretty efficiently every four hours, too. The second night was a little better and she's been on track ever since. I suggested that her parents keep her on the dream feed until six months, when they make the transition to solid food.

If a baby at this stage is still feeding every three hours, she might not be snacking, but I suspect that the parents are keeping her on an eating plan that's meant for a younger child. They need – gradually (by 15 minutes a day over a four-day period) – to lengthen the feeds to every four hours. Amuse them with toys and silly faces, or a walk in the park when they're hungry.

In a similar vein, parents who are worried that their baby is finishing his feeds 'too quickly' may be forgetting that their baby is growing up. Your baby may be getting plenty to eat but it just takes him less time to down it as he's now a more efficient eater. This, of course, depends on whether he's taking breast milk, which we measure in time, or formula, which is measured in ml/ounces.

If he's on formula, he should be taking between 150 and 250 ml (5 and 8 ounces) per feed, *every 4 hours.* Including a dream feed at night, he will therefore be taking a total of 775 to 1,100 ml (26 to 38 ounces) per day.

If he is a breastfed baby, feeds at this stage should only take around 20 minutes, because he's now able to consume in that short time the same 150 to 175 ml (5 or 6 ounces) of breast milk that once took him 45 minutes to finish. If you want to be sure, though, do a yield (page 52).

In either case, if your baby is nearing the six-month mark, it's time to introduce solids as well, because, as your baby begins to really move about, he needs more than just liquid to sustain his activities (see page 109).

As for the baby who 'doesn't seem interested' in feeds any more, I'm afraid that just goes with the territory. Between four and six months, your baby will be more curious and more mobile. She can turn her head and reach for things, so now eating is not necessarily a high priority. You may even have a week or two when she's absolutely uncooperative and impossible.

Take some proactive steps:

- Feed her in an area relatively free of distractions.

- Tuck her little arm in under you, so she doesn't start fiddling.

- If your baby is very active, you can half-swaddle her to cut down on the squirming.

- Put a brightly coloured piece of cloth that has decorations on it over your shoulder so your baby has something novel to look at.

Sometimes, I have to admit, the best you can do is ride it out – and watch in awe at what a little person your baby is becoming.

CHAPTER SIX
Getting Ready

Four to Six Months

Somewhere around four months, when many parents start thinking about giving their child solid foods, it's not necessarily a problem, more a set of concerns:

> *When should we start solids?*
> *What foods should we try?*
> *How will we get our baby to chew?*
> *What's the proper way to feed him?*

Most of those questions are a matter of readiness. Babies are born with a tongue-thrust reflex that initially helps them latch on to a nipple and suck effectively. When this instinctive protrusion of the tongue disappears, somewhere between four and six months, babies are then able to swallow thick, mushy foods, like cereal and pureed fruits and vegetables.

Solid Advice

Sometimes paediatricians advocate adding solids for reflux babies, reasoning that heavier foods are more likely to stay in the stomach. In such cases, I advise clients to seek the help of a gastroenterologist, who can determine if their baby's intestines are mature enough to handle solid food. Otherwise, the baby might get constipated, and you'll just be exchanging one gastric problem for another.

Your baby is probably not ready at four months. The current Department of Health guideline is to start solids at six months and I (and many paediatricians) believe that it's best to be on the conservative side and start solids at around six months; before that, babies' digestive systems aren't mature enough to metabolise solid foods. Most are also not able to sit upright, and it's more challenging for them to take in solids while reclining. In addition, allergies are more likely to develop in younger babies, so it makes sense to play it safe.

Earlier than Six Months

If you're thinking about giving solids earlier, ask yourself these questions to see if your child is getting ready to start solids:

Does my baby seem hungrier than usual? Unless he's been sick or has been teething (see pages 128–129), increased feeds often indicate that a baby needs more than an all-liquid diet supplies. Every day, the average four-to-six-month-old consumes around 950–1075 ml (32–36 ounces) of breast milk or formula. For a large, active baby, especially one whose physical development is proceeding at a rapid pace, liquid alone might not be enough to sustain him.

In my experience with average-weight babies, activity only becomes a factor at five or six months. But if your baby is above average – for example, at four months weighs 7¼–7½ kg (16 or 17 pounds) – he drinks to full capacity at every meal, and still seems to need more nourishment, then it might be time to consider solids.

Does your baby get up in the middle of the night for a bottle? If your baby finishes a full bottle when she wakes, her night waking is due to hunger. But a four-month-old should not be eating in the middle of the night, so you first have to take steps to stop the night feedings (see page 74). Once you've upped her liquid intake *during the day*, if she still seems hungry for more, that might indicate that she needs solids as well.

It's a Myth

No scientific research supports the popular notion that solids help a baby sleep longer. A full tummy does help a baby sleep, but it doesn't have to be full of cereal. Breast milk or formula does the trick without running the risk of digestive problems or allergies.

Spotlight in the Trenches

Jack weighed 8 kg (18 pounds) at 4 months, and his parents were large, too – his mum was 1.75 m (5'9") and Dad, 2 m (6'5"). Jack was wolfing down 250 ml (8 ounces) of formula every 4 hours and had recently started waking in the

Spotlight in the Trenches *Cont'd*

night, too, always taking a full bottle. Although he was drinking nearly 200 ml (40 ounces) a day, his tummy could only hold so much liquid, and it was obviously not sustaining him.

I've seen this pattern in other babies, too. But instead of waking in the night, they seem hungry 3 hours after a full feed. Rather than keep a baby on a 3-hour routine, which is not appropriate for a 4-month-old, we introduce solids.

In either instance, if you start your child on solids as early as 4 months, the food has to be finely pureed. Most importantly, solids should be an add-on, not a replacement for breast milk or formula, as they are with children over 6 months.

Has your baby lost his tongue-thrust reflex? The tongue-thrust reflex is apparent when a baby roots or sticks his tongue out in search for food. This action helps babies suckle in infancy, but tongue-thrusting works against ingesting solid foods. Put a spoon into your baby's mouth: if the tongue-thrust reflex hasn't disappeared, his little tongue will automatically push the spoon out. Even when this reflex disappears, your baby will still need time to get used to eating from a spoon; at first, he'll probably try to suck it the way he sucked a nipple.

Does your baby look at you when you're eating as if to say, 'Hey, why aren't I getting any of that?' As young as four months, some babies start to notice us eating; most do by the time they're six months. Some even imitate a chewing motion. That's often the time parents decide to take those cues seriously and offer a few teaspoons of mushy food.

Can your baby sit up without support? It's best for a baby to have fairly good control of her neck and back muscles before starting solid food. Start your child out in an infant seat and then progress to a high chair.

Does your baby reach for things and put them in his mouth? Those are precisely the skills he'll need for finger foods.

Chapter Seven

Food Is More than Nourishment

Solid Foods

For the first few months after they're born, babies' taste buds aren't developed. Their liquid diet is bland, consisting of formula or breast milk, either of which provides them with all the nutrients they require. At no other time in your child's life will she gain weight at this rapid pace. And a good thing, too!

It takes a while to get into a good rhythm, but most parents eventually find that feeding a baby is relatively uncomplicated. Then, at around six months – just as you're beginning to feel comfortable with your baby's liquid diet – it's time to introduce solid foods. It doesn't happen overnight, but if you approach this period with a positive attitude and lots of patience, it can be fun to observe your baby as she experiments with each new food and makes – often fumbling – attempts to feed herself.

Terminology

In England, the transition from breast or bottle to solid food is described as 'weaning'. In the United States, 'weaning' only refers to getting off the breast or bottle – which may or may not happen around the same time you 'introduce' solid food. So here we'll talk about the two as separate processes.

Weaning and introducing solids are related: both are signs that your child is growing up. As your baby has become physically stronger and better coordinated, she has begun to squirm, turn her head, push a breast or bottle away; by six months, when she can sit up fairly well and is beginning to grab hold of things – a spoon, her bottle, your breast – it becomes obvious that she wants to be more of a partner in this eating thing.

You might welcome these changes, or they might make you sad. Many mums I've met have mixed feelings, or are downright distraught, and some even wait to introduce solids because they don't want to 'rush' the process. These are understandable feelings, but you need to let go and let your baby become an independent eater. Granted, she will have to work even harder at getting it right than she did as a tiny infant – and you'll have to have even more patience. But the payoff is having a child who relishes eating, is willing to experiment and associates food with good feelings.

From Feeding to Eating: The Adventure Continues

This at-a-glance chart shows the progression from feeding to eating, the basics of getting there and common concerns.

Age	Intake	Suggested schedule	Common concerns
Birth to 6 weeks (see page 41 for details)	85 ml (3 ounces) liquid	Every 2 to 3 hours, depending on baby's birthweight	Sleeping during feeds and hungry an hour later. Eating every 2 hours. Lots of rooting, but baby only takes a little bit at each feed. Crying during feeds or shortly thereafter.
6 weeks to 4 months (see page 41 for details)	125–150 ml (4–5 ounces) liquid	Every 3 to 3½ hours	Waking for night-time feeds (seemingly a sleep problem, it's cured by proper food management).
4–6 months (see page 42 for details)	175–250 ml (6–8 ounces) liquid If you start solids this early, place your baby in an infant seat or feed her on your lap, elevating her head. Solids should be finely pureed and almost watery at this age.	Every 4 hours If you start solids at this age, which I don't normally advise, liquids should still be the mainstay of your baby's diet.	Finishing bottle or breast too quickly – is she getting enough to eat? When to start solid foods? What foods should we try? How will we get our baby to chew?

Age	Intake	Suggested schedule	Common concerns
4–6 months (see page 42 for details) *Cont'd*	Restrict solids to pureed pears, apples, and single-grain baby cereals (not wheat), which are easiest to digest. Give 1–2 tsp. before the bottle or breast.		What's the proper way to feed her?
6–12 months	Everything will be pureed at first. Start with 1–2 tsp. for the 1st week, only at breakfast; the 2nd week, at breakfast and lunch; and the 3rd week, all 3 meals. You will add a new food every week – always at breakfast – and move the proven foods to lunch and dinner. Give solids when your child is alert and fully awake. If at first she finds it frustrating, take the edge off her hunger with a bit of breast or bottle. Once she gets the hang of things, always give solid foods first. As your baby adjusts and seems able to chew, add foods with some texture. Gradually progress to 25–40 g (1–1½ ounces) of solid per meal, more or less depending on her appetite and capacity. Finger foods are added at 9 months or when she can sit on her own.	It takes 2 months, at most 4, to ease into solids. By 9 months, most babies are eating solids at breakfast (approximately 9am), lunch (12 or 1pm), and dinner (5–6pm). Breast or bottle first thing in the morning, between feeds (as a snack), and before bed. By the end of the 1st year, you have gradually cut in half the amount of liquids you give as the amount of solids increases, so that solids are the mainstay of the diet. Your baby will drink between 475 and 950 ml (16 and 32 ounces) of liquid a day, depending on his size. Once he is able to eat finger foods, always start the meal with them and then spoon-feed other foods.	What solids to start with and how to introduce them? How much to feed compared with liquids? Having trouble adapting to solid foods (closing his lips so Mum can't even get the spoon in; gagging; choking). Fear of food allergies.1–2 years.

Age	Intake	Suggested schedule	Common concerns
6–12 months *Cont'd*	Suggested foods at 6–9 months: mild fruits and veg (apples, pears, peaches, plums, bananas; squash, sweet potatoes, carrots, green beans, peas); single-grain cereals; brown rice, bagels, chicken, turkey, cooked white fish (like cod), tinned tuna. By 9 months, start finger foods. You can also add pasta, stronger fruits (prunes, kiwi, pink grapefruit) and veg (avocado, asparagus, courgettes, broccoli, beetroot, potatoes, parsnips, spinach, butter beans, aubergine), beef broth, lamb. If you or your partner have allergies, consult with your doctor about the introduction of new foods.	At around 9 months, you can start giving light snacks between meals – bagel, biscuits, bits of cheese – but be careful not to let him fill up on snacks (see pages 125–127).	
1–2 years	Foods are no longer pureed; your toddler should be eating lots of finger foods and starting to feed himself. Once every week, you can also start introducing foods that are on my 'proceed with caution' list, such as dairy products, including yoghurt,	Three meals a day; bottle or breast morning and night until your child is completely weaned, usually by 18 months if not sooner. You can give light healthful snacks between meals, as long as it doesn't affect	Not eating as much as she used to. Still prefers his bottle to solid foods. Refuses to eat _____ [insert name of food, like carrots]. Refuses to wear bib.

Age	Intake	Suggested schedule	Common concerns
1–2 years *Cont'd*	cheese and cows' milk (see page 123), as well as whole eggs, honey, beef, melon, berries, citrus fruits other than pink grapefruit, lentils, pork and veal. I'd still be very careful with, even keep away from, nuts, which are hard to digest and easy to choke on, as well as shellfish and chocolate, because they can cause allergies.	your child's appetite for other foods. Plan at least one of your own meals around your toddler and pull her high chair up to the table, so she begins to get used to the idea of family dining.	Won't sit in the high chair or tries to climb out. Won't even try to feed herself. Mealtimes are a disaster – and a huge mess. Dumps or drops food.
2–3 years	By 18 months, and certainly by 2, your child should be eating a full range of foods, unless she has developed allergies or any other problems along the way. How much she eats depends on her size and appetite – some kids eat and need less than others. Your child should be eating what the family eats; resist the temptation to prepare a different dinner for her.	Three meals a day, with light snacks between meals. By now your child has very definite likes and dislikes, maybe even a sweet tooth. Resist giving too many snacks between meals, or snacks with little nutritional value or too much sugar. It will affect her intake at meals. For one meal of the day, at least a few days of the week, have family dinners so that your child becomes a social eater as well as a well-nourished human being.	Picky eating – not a 'good' eater. Food fads (eats same foods over and over). Quirky 'rules' around eating (cries if food breaks, peas and potatoes can't touch, etc.) Eats only snacks. Won't sit at dinner table. Atrocious manners. Throws food. Purposely makes mess. Has tantrums at mealtimes.

Food Management: Did You Grow Up in a B.A.R.N.?

Food management – making sure your child gets enough to eat, at the right times, and in the right amounts – is critical from the day he is born. When solid foods are added, though, good food management is once again essential.

With older children, there are four keys to food management: *Behaviour* (your child's), *Attitude* (yours), *Routine* and *Nourishment*. Most of the eating problems I encounter are related to one, if not more, of those elements.

Behaviour: Every family has a set of values that relate to eating; each has its own definition of what's proper. **When it comes to eating, what do you find acceptable and what won't you allow?** You have to figure out what *your* limits are and convey them.

Start when you first put your baby in a high chair. For instance, if you feel good table manners are important, your nine-month-old is not too young to learn. The moment he starts squashing or smearing his food, take him out of his high chair. Take his misbehaviour as a sign that he's finished eating and tell him, 'No, we do not play with our food. We sit at the table to *eat*.' He may not understand exactly what you are saying (or he might), but he will quickly make the association that the high chair is for eating not playing.

It's the same with manners. If you believe they're important, as I most certainly do, even before your child is old enough to say 'please' and 'thank you' and 'may I be excused from the table?' you say the words *for* her. If at home a child is allowed to climb out of her chair or put her feet on the eating tray, what do you expect her to do outside the home?

Attitude: Children imitate us. **Is food important to you? Do you care about the meals you serve and relish eating?** Maybe you mix everything together, you're always eating on the run or you serve utterly bland food. Or let's say you're always dieting and hyper-vigilant about what you eat. I've seen mothers put babies on a low-fat regimen or worry because their toddler is 'eating too many carbohydrates'. Both are nutritionally unsound; babies and toddlers have different food requirements from adults. Also, withholding food or labelling certain foods as 'bad' can send a message to your child that can later lead to serious eating issues.

Let children learn from experience. If you're always wiping your toddler's mouth or making comments about what a 'mess' he's making, your child will very quickly begin to view eating as an unpleasant experience.

Routine: I know you're sick of hearing the word 'routine', but being consistent about when and where a child eats, rather than eating on the go, tells your child that not only is eating important, but so is he. Make mealtime a priority, and, if it's at all possible, have family dinners together at least two nights a week. Be consistent, also, in the words you use. For example, if he goes to grab a slice of bread, you stop him and show him what to say: 'Please, may I have that?' If you do it every time, by the time he can say the words himself, he'll know what is expected of him.

Nourishment: Though we can't influence a child's capacity or appetite (except genetically), *choice* of food is controlled, at least in these early years, by parents. Your child may have particular or even peculiar tastes, but in the end it's up to you to ensure that he has healthy options. If you're an observant, healthy eater yourself, you'll probably have no trouble figuring out what to give your baby. But if you're not, please educate yourself about good nutrition so that when he gets to the point, usually around age two, that he's eating everything you eat, you won't be compromising your child's nutrition. Keeping a food log can be helpful because it will make you more conscious of what you're serving.

I also want to stress that your child will have good eating days and days when he couldn't care less about food. He might really love a particular food for a month and then suddenly refuse it. Or he might surprise you and eat something you've been trying to get him to taste for months. But don't insist and please don't get upset. Just keep giving him options.

> While he doesn't each much quantity-wise at a meal, 19-month-old Dexter will eat just about anything – and I know this is because we have given him all sorts of foods from the very beginning. We just offered whatever we were eating and he could choose to eat it or not. One example is broccoli; he hated the jarred baby broccoli, hated it the first 20 times I put it on his plate (he would sometimes try a nibble, sometimes not), then one day he just ate it and now Dexter loves it.
>
> We also don't make a big deal out of eating things. We don't say 'good boy for eating your cucumber', or 'if you eat your cabbage you will get a cookie', because that implies that there is something wrong or yucky with it, like it is a chore to be rewarded.
>
> Offer new foods! You would be amazed what toddlers will take a liking to!

Keep the B.A.R.N. keys – **B**ehaviour, **A**ttitude, **R**outine and **N**ourishment – in mind as you read through the following sections on what typically happens at each stage of your child's development and the common complaints that crop up. As always, I urge you to read through *all* the age-related sections, as some challenges that happen to a particular child at six months might come up for another child at a year.

CHAPTER EIGHT

Troublesome Transitions

Breast to Bottle/Bottle to Cup

Talk about giant steps! Your baby is about to enter the real world, at least when it comes to food. Well, almost. No more living solely on a liquid diet. Now he's going to learn how to eat mush and then little pieces and finally all the foods you eat.

I also suggest cutting out the dream feed at around seven months (see box, pages 96–97), as your baby starts to get solid food in him. If you continue to give it, you're working against the introduction of solid food because, for every 25 ml/ounce of extra liquid your baby takes, he won't be hungry for 25 grams/an ounce of solid food. However, when you cut out the dream feed, ensure you add the same number of ml or grams or ounces to the day feed; otherwise, your baby will wake up at night.

How Do I Stop the Dream Feeds?

The process of cutting out the dream feed – usually at around 7 months – has to be done in 3-day increments, to ensure that during the day your baby makes up for what you're taking away at night:

Day 1: Add 25 ml (1 ounce) to the first feed of the day, and take away 25 ml (1 ounce) from the dream feed that night. If you're breastfeeding, go back to clustering so that you get more calories in. Give the dream feed (now 25 ml/1 ounce less) half an hour earlier, at 10.30 instead of 11.

Day 4: Add 25 ml (1 ounce) to the first feed, 25 ml (1 ounce) to the second, and take away

The other most common concerns at this stage are:

> *My baby still wakes up hungry at night.*
> *I'm trying to get my baby on a bottle, but she's having none of it.*
> *My baby uses a trainer cup but she won't drink milk out of it.*

Like many problems that crop up after the six-month mark, these are most likely the result of accidental parenting. Take the first one: when a baby is still waking up for food at six months it's because parents have responded to earlier episodes of night waking with a feed, even though the baby only took a few ml/ounces.

When babies night wake at different times, it is usually hunger but, by six months, I rarely see this, except during growth spurts or when it's time to introduce solids. But when they wake up like clockwork, it's usually about accidental parenting. Hold them off by using my pick-up/put-down method. The good news? It takes less time with older babies to change this habit because they have enough fat on their bodies to last between feeds.

The second and third complaints are also due to accidental parenting. If parents don't introduce a bottle early (see page 98), three, six or ten months later, I often get frantic calls: 'I'm a prisoner, because no one else can feed her' or 'My husband thinks our baby hates him because she screams if he tries to give her a bottle'.

It's the same with making the transition to a trainer cup. This is a common scenario: a mum will introduce her baby to this more grown-up form of drinking by giving him something other than breast milk or formula. Often it's juice, because he'll be more

> ## How Do I Stop the Dream Feeds? *Cont'd*
>
> 50 ml (2 ounces) from the dream feed. Give the dream feed (50 ml/2 ounces less) at 10.
>
> *Day 7:* Add 25 ml (1 ounce) to the first feed, 25 ml (1 ounce) to the second, 25 ml (1 ounce) to the third, take away 75 ml (3 ounces) from the dream feed, and give it at 9.30.
>
> *Days 10* (dream feed at 9pm), *14* (8.30), *17* (8.00) and *20* (7.30): By continuing every 3 days to add 25 ml (1 ounce) during the day, and taking away the same amount from the dream feed, you will end up doing a feed at 7.30 with only a few ounces.

willing to drink the sweet, strange-tasting liquid from a cup than boring old milk, or water. Then, after a few months of

Winding Down Breastfeeding

Whether they want to quit altogether or just wind down, many mothers are worried about how their breasts will feel when they first skip a feed. This plan assumes that your baby is willing to take a bottle and that you want to continue breastfeeding only twice a day, in the morning and after work. If you want to quit altogether, just keep eliminating feeds. Your body will cooperate, but you have to help it along.

Pump instead of skipping feeds. To avoid becoming engorged, for 12 days continue to put your baby on your breasts in the morning and whenever you want to give the second feed. During the day, pump when you'd normally feed him. Pump 15 minutes per session for the first three days. On the fourth, fifth

tasting that 'other' liquid, when Mum tries to give him milk instead, he thinks 'This isn't supposed to be in *here*' and he categorically refuses to drink it. (See page 106 for what to do.)

From Breast to Bottle: The First Steps of Weaning

There are two factors that influence what happens when you try to introduce a bottle: your baby's reaction and yours (both emotional and physical). You might want to introduce a bottle because you're ready to wean your baby entirely, or because you want to make your life easier by replacing one or more breastfeeding sessions with bottle-feeds. The older your baby, the harder it will be for you to get her used to a bottle in the first place if she's been exclusively on the breast. But, with older babies, it will also be easier for your body to adapt to the change, because your milk will dry up more quickly (see box). At the same time, though, a lot of mums have a strong emotional reaction to reducing the number of breastfeeds and, especially, to quitting altogether.

The procedure for the baby is the same for one who's never had a bottle as it is for one who had one several months earlier and now seems to have forgotten how to drink from one. Regardless of whether you're switching to a bottle and plan never to breastfeed again or you want to do only a few feeds a day, my advice is to make sure you're ready, stay the course, and steel yourself for a bumpy day or two. (Of course, if your baby is six months or older, you might consider going straight to a trainer cup and skip the bottle.)

Find a type of nipple that most closely resembles your own. Some gung-ho breastfeeding experts warn of 'nipple

Winding Down Breastfeeding
cont'd

and sixth days, pump only 10 minutes. On the seventh, eighth and ninth, 5 minutes. And on the last three days, only 2 to 3 minutes. By then, your breasts will fill only before the two feeds, and you won't need to continue pumping.

Wear a tight bra between feeds. A snug sports bra helps your body reabsorb the milk.

Do 3 to 5 sets of overarm exercises daily. Act as if you're throwing a ball. This also aids reabsorption. If necessary, take a painkiller every 4 to 6 hours for pain. Engorgement is rare when a baby is 8 months or older; milk production stops more quickly than at, say, 3 months.

confusion' but, if anything, babies can be confused by *flow*, not the nipple itself. If your baby takes to a certain type, don't keep switching – *unless* she starts choking, spluttering or gagging. If so, buy the slow-release type of nipple, which is specially designed to respond to her suckling actions, as opposed to the standard types, which drip into her mouth even when she stops sucking.

Start with the first bottle of your baby's day, when she's hungriest. What's her incentive to accept the bottle if not hunger? But still expect that your baby will be resistant and ill at ease.

Never force the bottle. Imagine what it is like after several months of sucking on warm, human flesh to taste a cold rubber nipple for the first time. To make it more like your body temperature, run warm water over it. Push it into his mouth gently and jiggle it on his bottom lip, which stimulates the sucking reflex. If he doesn't take it within five minutes, stop, or you'll give him an aversion to it. Wait an hour and try again.

Try every hour the first day. Be persistent. Any mum who says she's been at it for 12 weeks, or even four weeks, is not really keeping at it. More likely, she tries for a day or two – or even a few minutes – and then again only when she starts feeling tied down once more. If she doesn't commit to staying with it every day, it's less likely to work.

Let Dad or a friend give it a try, but only when you're first introducing the bottle. Some babies take bottles from others and absolutely refuse it from their mums. It's a good way to get your baby started, but it's not something you want to foster. Once she's accustomed to the bottle, you give it to her, too.

Expect – and be willing to ride out – a hunger strike. If your baby refuses the bottle altogether, don't whip out your breast. I promise, your child won't starve to death. Most babies will take at least some food after three or four hours of not getting the breast. I've seen babies refuse bottles all day long, but those are the exceptions (and they don't starve either). If you're persistent, the trauma of introducing a bottle is usually over within 24 hours (and two or three days for some older babies).

Thereafter, always give a bottle at least once a day. A common mistake that mothers make is not sticking with at least a once-a-day bottle. Babies will always go back to their original

Making the Switch

Janna had been leaving work every day in order to feed her seven-month-old baby Justin. Now she really wanted to have the flexibility of a bottle. At my suggestion, she gave Justin a feed before she left for work and left a bottle of pumped milk for the nanny to do the midday feed. But Justin refused and went on a hunger strike. Every time Janna called home, she heard Justin crying in the background: 'I thought he was starving. I don't think I've ever suffered through a day as much as that one.'

When Janna arrived home at four, Justin was still screaming for her breast. She offered him a bottle instead and, when he pitched a fit, told him calmly, 'Okay, you're not hungry now.' By six he was willing to take the bottle.

feeding method, but they won't remember the second method you teach them unless you keep it up. If you do let it lapse, start again, using the method above to *re*introduce the bottle.

'But My Baby . . .': Mums' Feelings of Loss and Guilt over Weaning

There's one other piece of advice I have about taking steps to begin the weaning process: make sure you *want* to introduce a bottle. In Janna's case (see box), for example, her fears about Justin starving were not merely about his physical well-being. She was feeling guilty for causing him to 'suffer' and, I would wager, ambivalent about the whole process.

Looking at my website recently, I came across a series of postings in response to a mother who for nine months had had trouble keeping up her supply and getting her son to nurse. Determined to 'make it at least a year', she felt guilty for 'wanting a little freedom' and wondered if 'anyone ever felt like this?' If she only knew. Here's a sampling of the comments from the mums who responded:

> 'Ultimately, it is your decision. You know what is best for you and your child.'

> 'Nine months is wonderful. It is a major commitment to nurse for any period of time and I commend the mothers who attempt it for even a short amount of time.'

> 'I had a mixed bag of emotions, too. On the one hand, I wanted to continue nursing for as long as possible. On the other, I wanted my freedom and own identity. I wanted to be Rosa and not just Marina's Lactating Mother. When I did wean, I missed our closeness. However, I gained my normal breasts back. I didn't have to worry about leaking. I no longer had to use a bra at night for sleeping. And DH was no longer restricted from that zone!'

Breastfeeding is a wonderful experience for some mothers, and I'm all for it. But there comes a time for it to end. Perhaps it

Making the Switch *cont'd*

Janna called me afterwards and said, 'I'd like to breastfeed him tonight.' I told her she couldn't unless she wanted another hunger strike the following day. She had to keep up the bottles for two days before she could resume giving him the bedtime feed.

Too Old for a Bottle?

Mothers are often advised to get rid of the bottle by a year or 18 months at the latest, but I think two is plenty of time. It's not the end of the world if your baby takes a few minutes at bedtime with his bottle to snuggle up in Mum or Dad's lap.

Left to their own devices, many toddlers give up their bottles voluntarily by the age of two. When they want to hang on longer it's usually because they've been allowed to use a bottle as a 'dummy' to keep him happy, or the parents may use a bottle to send him off to naps or night-time sleep. Some parents leave a bottle in the child's cot, hoping to grab an extra hour of sleep, which is not only habit-forming, it's dangerous – the child could choke. Also,

will ease your guilt to know that you're not weaning just because you're tired of leaky breasts or pumping at work, but for the sake of your baby's growing up and moving on to the next stage.

Trainer Cups: I'm a Big Kid Now!

Around the time you start thinking about introducing solid food, you should also think about getting your child used to a trainer cup, so that he can make the transition from sucking his liquids down through a nipple to drinking like the big kids. It, too, is part of allowing your child to grow up, to go from being fed to eating on his own (and some breast-feeding mums go straight from breast to trainer cup).

When a mother says to me, 'I just can't get my child to use a trainer cup', I ask my questions:

At what age did you first try to introduce it? Even if a baby is on a bottle and breast, at six months it's important to try out a trainer cup (which is better than a plastic cup, in that it has a spout that controls the flow). Your child can hold it herself, which promotes her independence. (Never *ever* give a glass to a baby or young child, not even up to four or five years old.)

How often did you try to give it? You have to give your child three weeks to a month of *daily* practice for him to get used to a trainer cup. It will take longer if you don't give it every day.

Did you try different types? Few babies immediately take to a trainer cup. If yours doesn't like it at first, remember that it's new and foreign to him. Breastfeeding babies often do better with a straw type of trainer cup rather than those with a spout but, regardless of the type you buy, stick with one type for at least a month. Resist switching from one to another.

Too Old for a Bottle? *Cont'd*

when a child is allowed to nurse a bottle all day, he fills up on liquid and often eats less food.

If your child is two or older, it's time to intervene:

- Make some ground rules about the bottle – only at bedtime or only in the bedroom.
- Bring snacks with you, instead of relying on the bottle for sustenance.
- Make the bottle less attractive. Cut a slit in the nipple, about 6–9 mm (¼–½ inch) across. Wait 4 days and then cut a slit the other way, so you have an X. After another week, cut first 2 and then all 4 of the triangles. Eventually, you'll have a big square opening and your child will lose interest altogether.

How Much Fluid a Day?

Once your child is on solid food three times a day, he should be having at least 475 ml (16 ounces) of milk or formula a day (up to 950 ml/32 ounces for big babies). Most mums split it up and give a little liquid after meals to wash down food and also offer a thirst-quencher after they've been running around.

Don't wean if your child is solely on breast milk until he's mastered a trainer cup or at least is willing to drink from a bottle.

In what position do you hold your baby when giving him a trainer cup? Sit your baby on your knee, facing outwards. Guide his little hands on to the handles and help him pick the cup up to his mouth. Do it gently, and do it at a time when he's in a good mood.

How much – and what kind of – liquid do you put into the cup? Too much liquid will mean that the trainer cup is too heavy for the baby to hold. I'd recommend no more than 25 ml (an ounce) of water, pumped milk or formula to begin with. Avoid juice, because your baby doesn't need the extra sugar (and she may always associate the trainer cup with a sweet liquid and refuse all others).

If you have already made that mistake and she's now using a trainer cup like a champ but refuses to drink milk in it, you can't go cold turkey on her – she'll get upset, perhaps start associating the trainer cup with a negative experience, and she might even get dehydrated (especially if she's been weaned from the breast and doesn't take a bottle). Start by offering her two cups of liquid at her meal. In one, have 25 ml (an ounce) of the liquid you've been giving her – say juice or water – and in the other pour 50 ml (2 ounces) of milk. After she has a sip of the water, take that cup away and try to give her the milk. If she refuses, leave it and try an hour later. Even if she's already proficient, try sitting her on your knee for a drink. As with most things, if you persist, and don't see it as a skill you have to teach her *immediately*, you're more likely to be successful.

CHAPTER NINE

Help! We Need a Solid-food Consultant!

Six to Twelve Months

Most babies are ready to begin eating solids in earnest at this age, and it is the prime time. Because they're more active now, even 950 ml (32 ounces) or more of breast milk or formula isn't enough to keep them going. The process will take a few months, but gradually your child will develop a pattern of eating three solid meals a day. He will continue to have breast- or bottle-feeds in the morning, between meals, and at night. By eight or nine months, you will have introduced several types of foods – cereal, fruit and vegetables, chicken, fish – and your baby should be well on his way to being a good eater of solid foods. By a year, solids will replace half his liquid intake.

At around the same time, your baby's manual dexterity will take a giant leap, which means he can coordinate his little fingers and use them like pincers to pick up small objects.

Ideally, you want to encourage him to use this newfound skill to pick up finger foods (see box, pages 116–118).

This six-month period is probably the most exciting and, to some mums, the most frustrating time because it's all about trial and error. Your baby is tasting new foods and learning to chew – or gum – them. Once he starts picking up finger foods, he'll need to develop the coordination to find his mouth and actually get food into it. At first, more will end up in his ears and hair, as well as on his bib or on the floor. This is also the time I get calls from confused parents:

> *I don't know where to begin – what food to start with, or how to do it.*
> *How much solid food do I feed now, compared with liquids?*
> *When I look at charts in various books, I'm afraid my child isn't eating enough.*
> *My baby is having trouble adapting to solid foods.*
> *I'm worried about food allergies, which I hear are common in babies who are on solids.*

The important thing to remember is that, at this stage, almost everyone has some type of confusion, so you're not alone. Also, it's much easier to correct problems now before bad habits – your child's and yours – have a chance to develop.

At what age did you begin to introduce solids? I often get calls from parents of six-, seven-, or even eight-month olds, who had been started earlier than my advised six months – say at four months (see Chapter 6). Things went smoothly for a while, but then the baby began to refuse solids. Often, but not always, this coincides with teething, a cold or any other vulnerable time in the baby's life. In most of these cases, as the parents introduced solids, they also decreased their baby's suckling time. And when a baby is deprived of suckling time in this way, essentially weaning him too early, there's a good chance he'll want to make up for it and demand more of the bottle or breast.

Be patient, and keep offering the solids. Continue to give him the bottle or breast. If you're relaxed about it, his reluctance should last no more than a week to 10 days. Never force solid foods, but if he still seems hungry *do not feed him in the night*; keep offering solids during the day. If he's hungry, he'll eventually try them.

Was your baby premature? If so, even six months might be too early to introduce solids. Remember that her chronological age, counting from the day she was born, is not the same as her developmental age, which determines readiness, and her digestive system might not be ready for solids. Go back to the liquid diet, and at seven and a half or eight months, try again.

What is your baby's temperament? Think of how your baby has been with other new circumstances and transitions. Temperament always influences how he reacts to his environment, including how well he adapts to new foods. Modify your introduction of solids accordingly. **How long have you been trying to introduce solids?** It could be that your expectations are too high. Imagine, after having solely breast milk or formula, what it must be like to feel a sloppy mass in your mouth. Some children can take as long as two or three months to get used to the idea of 'chewing' down solids. Stay with it and remain calm yourself.

What are you feeding your baby? Introducing solid foods is a gradual process of going from very sloppy and runny foods at first to finger foods. I recommend starting with fruit; pears are easy to digest and fruit has more nutritional value than cereal. Few babies take any kind of solid straight away. You have to start with one teaspoon and you may have to try many times; the process is very slow and gradual:

- For the first two weeks, give only one to two teaspoons of pears at breakfast and at dinner, and continue to give bottle or breast when your baby wakes up, at lunch, and before bed.

- Assuming your baby has no adverse reaction, introduce a second food, such as squash, again giving the new food at breakfast and moving the pears to dinner.

- Try out a new vegetable or fruit – sweet potatoes or apple in the third week – in the morning.

- By the fourth week, you can introduce oatmeal and give your baby solids at lunch as well, increasing the amount to three or four teaspoons per meal, more or less depending on your baby's weight and capacity.

- In the next four weeks, you can add rice or barley cereal, peaches, bananas, carrots, peas, green beans, sweet potatoes, plums.

Shop-bought food or home-made?

Either. When you're doing potato and veg for the whole family, puree them for your baby. Remember that you're trying to help your baby's taste buds blossom – don't mix everything together. That doesn't mean you shouldn't add a bit of apple sauce to his cereal to make it more appealing, but you're feeding a child, not a dog.

If you want to make your own baby food, be sure to ask yourself, 'How much time am I willing – and do I need – to invest?' If you don't have the time, don't panic. The mush stage

How Much Solid Food Equals One Ounce of Liquid?

1 ice cube = 25 g (1 ounce)
3 tsp = 1 T. = 12 g (½ ounce)
2 T. = 25 g (1 ounce)
1 jar of baby food = whatever weight it says on the label
Or, put another way:
2 T. of solid = 25 ml (1 ounce) of liquid
2 T. of solid fruit or veg mashed = ¼ of a 100 g (4-ounce) jar, if not making your own

lasts only a few months. It won't harm your baby to have some bottled foods. Moreover, even the big companies are now preparing organic baby foods with fewer additives; simply read the labels.

If you're one of those parents who worries whether your baby or toddler is getting 'enough', set aside a week to keep track. But how do you figure out what four spoonfuls each of apple sauce and oatmeal add up to in nutritional terms? You need to count grams/ounces (see box).

If you make your own baby food, freeze the food in ice-cube trays, which makes it easy to measure – one cube equals 25 g (one ounce) – and is more convenient. (If you use the microwave to thaw and reheat food, be careful; always stir and check the temperature before feeding it to your child.)

It's easier to gauge with shop-bought baby food, too. If your baby is eating a whole jar, simply look at the label to see how much he's eaten. If he eats only a half or quarter jar, pay attention to how many spoonfuls he eats and tally that up in grams/ounces.

You can do the same with finger foods. If, for example, you buy some turkey that weighs 100 grams (4 ounces) and there are four slices in the package, you know that each slice is 25 grams (1 ounce). You can compute the weight of cheese and most other finger foods in this way or at least come up with a good guesstimate.

This might sound complicated and like a lot of trouble, and I mostly suggest this to parents who are worried because their babies have lost more than 15 to 20 per cent of their weight (a little weight fluctuation is normal) or have lower than usual energy levels (in which case I also tell them to talk to their doctor or to a nutritionist).

The important thing is to give your child a balanced diet of fruits, vegetables, dairy, protein and whole grains. Remember that we're talking about tiny tummies here. One way to think about portion size is to give one to two tablespoons of food for each year of a child's life – at age one, one to two tablespoons; at age two, two to four; at age three, three to six. A 'meal' is usually two or three portions, but your child may eat far less or far more, depending on his size and appetite.

Fine Points of Finger Foods

When: At eight or nine months or when your baby is able to sit on his own in a high chair.

How: Don't pop it in his mouth for him, just put the food on the tray of his high chair. He might just smash it and spread it around; it's part of the learning experience. Eat some yourself. He will soon get the idea, especially if it's something yummy. Give finger foods first, before you start feeding him. If he doesn't eat them, don't worry about it. Just keep presenting them at the beginning of every meal, and he eventually will.

What: Sample it for yourself first – finger food should dissolve easily in your mouth and have no grit, grain or crumbs on which your baby could choke. Pretend you don't

Common problems at this stage

Does your baby reject the spoon? When introducing a spoon, take care to put the food on your baby's lips, just inside her mouth. If you stick the spoon too far in, it might cause her to gag. And just one or two instances of this might be enough for your child to associate the spoon with an unpleasant experience.

If your baby has no problem with the spoon, it won't be long before she tries to grab it out of your hands. Let her. Even playing with it will help her get ready for feeding herself. Have an arsenal of three or even four spoons on the ready: you feed her with one, allow her to grab it; use one in reserve; she'll probably drop a few as well.

Does your baby frequently gag or choke? If you're just starting to introduce solids, it could be because you're putting the spoon in too far (see above), putting too much on the spoon, or because you're rushing him – shovelling in another mouthful before he's had a chance to gum down the first. It could also be that the food isn't pureed enough. Whatever the reason, it won't take your baby very long to conclude they'd rather have a bottle.

Gagging also might be unrelated – some babies simply need more time to get used to the sensation of solids. If your baby gags or doesn't seem to enjoy his first tastes of solid foods, stop. Try again a few days later.

If your baby is past that initial stage, and you've started her on finger foods, she still might choke or gag once in a while, especially with an unfamiliar food. Don't introduce finger foods too early and be careful about what you give her.

Ellie is nearly six months so I am going to start giving her finger food. I was told to give her anything that will turn to mush easily, like small slices of dry toast, or baby rusks.

Fine Points of Finger Foods
cont'd

have any teeth and use your tongue to shove the food to the roof of your mouth and, with a series of jabs, squash it.

Be creative. Even oatmeal (cooked to a slightly stiffer consistency), mashed sweet or ordinary potatoes, or large-curd cottage cheese can be a finger food.

It depends on your tolerance for mess.

Ripe fruit is a great finger food, but sometimes it's better to cut it in larger chunks or sticks, because it tends to be slippery.

If your baby looks longingly at what you're eating (and it passes the above tests), let him try it. The more you allow your child to eat on his own, the more quickly he will learn, and the more he'll enjoy eating.

Fine Points of Finger Foods

cont'd

Here are a few suggestions:
• Cheerios or other dense, chunky dry cereals (avoid flakes at first)
• Pasta of various shapes – toss with pureed vegetables to add flavour and nutrition
• Baby chicken sausages
• Sliced pieces of chicken or turkey
• Tinned tuna or other kinds of cooked fish (left over from your dinner)
• Avocado chunks
• Semi-soft cheeses, like string cheese, soft Cheddar, Babybel
• 'Crazy sandwiches' – bread with crust cut off (can be shaped with a cookie cutter) and spread with sugarless jam, hummus, cream cheese or cottage cheese. Can also be grilled
• Bagel, plain or with any of above spreads

Well, that advice was right about the mush part, but not about the dry toast. First of all, dry toast has crumbs that little Ellie might inhale or catch in her throat. Second, six months is too early for most children to start finger foods. They need to be able to sit up without your help, which is usually not before eight or nine months. And it takes babies a month or two of getting used to the feeling of mushy solids in their mouth before attempting different textures. They have to practise pushing the food to the roof of their mouth and squishing it with their tongue until it turns to mush (see box).

Have you been consistent about giving your baby solid foods, or do you sometimes offer her your breast (or a bottle) because it's convenient or because you feel guilty? Whatever the reason for Mum's inconsistency, the problem is that children learn from repetition and by knowing what to expect. If you give your baby three meals of solid foods on some days, one or two on others, she is going to be confused. And then she will retreat to what she knows and what gives her comfort – suckling.

After eating, does your baby vomit, develop a rash, have diarrhoea or unusually loose stools? If so, what kinds of solids have you introduced and how often? He may be having some type of adverse reaction to a particular food, even an allergy. Although he won't make the connection between eating solids and not feeling well, a baby in pain or feeling under the weather won't be very eager to try new experiences.

Go very slowly. Start with *one* food, and one food only. For the first week (or 10 days, if your baby is on the sensitive side), give that food at the morning meal. Stick with that one food for a week, after which you can move it up to the midday meal and introduce another new food in the morning. As each new food passes this test, you can combine it with other foods you've already introduced.

I always suggest trying new foods in the morning so that, if a problem develops, it's less likely to upset your baby's night-time sleep and it's easier to determine the cause of your baby's distress.

If you have a baby with a sensitive system or allergies run in your family, you ought to be particularly vigilant. Paediatric allergies have increased over the last 20 years and *they don't get better by giving the child more of the triggering food – they get worse*. Keep a log of the foods you introduce and when so that, if your baby has frequent or serious reactions, you have the information when you consult your paediatrician.

CHAPTER TEN

Food Mismanagement and the Food Olympics

One to Two Years

The question 'How much should my child be eating?' becomes a bit tricky around the first birthday, both because babies come in all sizes and have different needs and because their rate of growth starts to slow at one year, they don't need quite as much fuel and their appetites naturally diminish. Don't panic. (Teething in the first year can also interfere with eating – see box, pages 128–129.)

At the same time, your child hopefully will have expanded her repertoire of foods. She should have tasted – and now be able to eat – a variety of solids, including finger foods. Some children just get to that point at a year; others have been eating solids since around nine months. But most are well on their way.

Your baby should now be having five feeds a day, three of mostly solids and two of around 250 ml (8 ounces) of liquid

Proper Fuel = Proper Weight Gain

At your baby's periodic visits, your doctor will check his health, weigh him, and make sure his gains are consistent with his age and size.

Report any changes in his energy level to the doctor. If your child is between one year and 18 months, low energy might indicate that he is not getting enough solids compared to liquids or that he's not eating foods that will fuel him. If he's older, he might not be eating enough protein to fuel his active lifestyle.

per feed for a total of 475 ml (16 ounces). In other words, half his liquid intake should be replaced by solids. If, however, he is still downing 950 ml (32 ounces) of breast milk, formula or cows' milk (see box, pages 123–124), you have to adjust that balance by decreasing the liquid and adding more solid food. If all goes as planned, at around 14 months, he will begin to develop the coordination needed to feed himself, a skill that continues to develop (with your help). Of course, things don't always go as planned. Problems at this stage fall into one of two categories: food mismanagement and the 'food Olympics' (see pages 127–134).

Food Mismanagement

When a child over one still prefers his bottle to solid foods, it usually indicates some form of food mismanagement, often an earlier issue. **At what age did you begin to introduce solids? What are you feeding your baby?**

How long have you been trying to introduce solids? Have you been consistent about giving your baby solid foods?

If you started too early you could be having the backlash reaction (see Chapter 9). If you recently started or if you haven't been consistent, you might need nothing more than a little patience. Although six months is a prime time, your baby might be taking a bit longer to adjust to solids. Just remember that the goal is to replace half the liquid intake with solids. So, add up what your child normally drinks in ounces at breakfast, lunch, and dinner, and then convert it into solids. For instance, if little Dominic usually has a 175 ml (6-ounce) bottle at breakfast, the idea is to get him to eat the equivalent in solid food – say 50 grams (2 ounces) of cereal, 50 grams (2 ounces) of fruit and 50 grams (2 ounces) of baby yoghurt (see page 114 for amounts).

Always give your baby solid food *first* at the three main meals of the day. Until he's weaned, which for most children is around

Milk

At one year, most paediatricians suggest making the transition from breast milk or formula to cows' milk, as well as introducing many of the 'proceed with caution' foods, like eggs and beef, to the diet, because the likelihood of developing allergies diminishes (unless other family members have them).

With milk, go slowly to make sure your baby doesn't have a reaction. Start by replacing the morning feed with whole milk. After a few days to a week (depending on your child's sensitivity and if your child has no reaction – diarrhoea, rash, vomiting), give him the milk in the afternoon and finally in the evening.

Milk *cont'd*

Some people like to introduce cows' milk by mixing it with breast milk or formula. I disagree – that way, if your baby has a reaction, how will you know whether it's because of the mixing or the milk itself?

18 months, his bottle or a breastfeed can be his 'snack' between meals. Once he's accustomed to eating solids, you can also offer your baby a trainer cup of water or milk to quench his thirst *after* the meal.

Sometimes the problem is not *all* solids but a particular kind of food – say, peaches. If your toddler isn't very adventurous about trying new foods or seems 'picky' and rejects certain foods, it's because children now start showing distinct preferences. It also might mean that he just needs a little more time to get used to the new flavours and sensations in his mouth.

Some children are, in fact, picky eaters – they don't like a big variety of foods at this stage and they never will. And some simply require less food than others. If a child doesn't want to eat all his food, allow him. Otherwise he can't learn when he's full. In my experience, if a baby is on a good routine, even a picky eater will try new solids. Just try two teaspoons of a new food – that way, you're at least introducing it to him.

My rule of thumb is to give a new food four days in a row. If your child doesn't eat it, give it a rest and try a week later. If your child doesn't like a huge variety of foods (see Food Fads on page 138), don't worry about it – some adults don't either. But I've found that when parents eat lots of different kinds of foods themselves, and expose their children to a variety of tastes without forcing the issue, their kids usually end up being fairly adventurous eaters. Also, don't be surprised if your child relishes sweet potatoes for two months and then suddenly doesn't like them. Just go with the flow.

> **Don't Pry**
>
> Trying to pry a 9- or 11-month-old's mouth open is like trying to get a fish from the jaws of a shark. If your child won't open her mouth for another bit, assume that she's finished eating and doesn't want any more.

Does your baby get up in the middle of the night to nurse or have a bottle? Liquid intake, especially night feeds, can interfere with a baby's desire to eat solid food. It's not rocket science: if your baby fills up on breast milk or formula, there's no room for solids! Also, by giving your baby a bottle or your breast in the middle of the night, even if he's hungry, you're inadvertently going backwards to a 24-hour routine.

Does your child eat a lot of snacks? If so, he might be filling himself up between meals. I'm not against giving a child a biscuit every now and then, but I do prefer more healthful snacks, like fruits or bits of cheese. Instead of making excuses when your child refuses to eat ('She's tired', 'She's getting new

From Snacker to Eater in 3 Days

When your child wakes at 7am, she'll have a bottle or feed.

At breakfast, around 9am, she'll have more of a snack than a full meal.

When her energy starts flagging at 10.30, instead of giving her biscuits, fruit or whatever is usual, distract her. Maybe take her out to play.

I guarantee that, by lunch, she'll eat more because she'll be very hungry. (If she's really out of sorts, make lunch a little earlier.)

In the afternoon, skip her usual snack after her nap. If she normally has a bottle when she wakes, halve the usual amount.

teeth'), take a proactive stance and eliminate giving so many filling snacks, especially those with empty calories (see box).

Snacks are a way of life once your baby starts to socialise, and the more he socialises, the more he will be exposed to a wide variety of snacks, including junk foods. Bring your own so you can control what he eats.

This is not to say that snacks are a bad thing. In fact, for some smaller-built children, they supply more calories than meals. Observe your child's eating patterns: if he has trouble finishing his meal and his weight is in a low percentile, it might be normal for him – some little tummies need to eat more often. It wouldn't hurt to give him more high-calorie snacks, like avocado, cheese, ice cream. Also, talk to your doctor about feeding him more often.

Do you take his not eating personally?
Under a year, not eating is rarely a matter of wilfulness or spite. So there's usually

something else going on, such as teething (see box, pages 128–129), lack of sleep, illness or it's simply not an eating day. But over a year, the act of not eating could be a weapon that your toddler has discovered he can use against you. If you have a great deal of anxiety around what he eats, I guarantee that, by 15 months or earlier, he will pick up on your feelings. In such cases, I've seen children refuse to try new foods or refuse to eat altogether.

> **From Snacker to Eater in 3 Days** Cont'd
>
> Remember that we're doing this at most for 3 days. You're not depriving her or starving her. It will be harder on you than her but, if you don't give in, by the third day, or often sooner, your baby will be eating full meals, not snacking.

The Food Olympics

Concerns that fall in this category include:

I have to chase my child around the kitchen to get him to eat.
My child won't sit in the high chair, or tries to climb out.
My child won't even try to feed herself.
My child refuses to wear a bib.
My child repeatedly drops food on the floor – or dumps it on his head.

Teething: An Appetite Buster

Signs (any or all of these):

Reddened cheeks

Nappy rash

Drooling

Gnawing on fingers

Runny nose and other signs of a postnasal drip

Fever

Concentrated urine

You put a bottle or breast in his mouth and he comes off it immediately because his gums are sore

His appetite may diminish because eating is so uncomfortable

If you touch the area on the gum, you may feel a bump or see a reddened spot

If you're breastfeeding you might feel the actual tooth coming through

Does your child often misbehave at mealtimes? Your child's newfound skills at the dinner table are happening at the same time as she's making huge developmental strides. Many children can walk at this age. Those who can't are at least crawling and climbing. And all are endlessly curious. Who wants to sit in a chair, even for 10 minutes, when there's a world out there to explore? And who wants to eat food, when throwing and smearing it are so much more fun?

In many households with one- to two-year-olds, mealtimes are trying, if not a disaster, and a huge mess. Parents' concerns reflect their toddler's growing independence, ability and, as he gets closer to age two, his wilfulness. In fact, sometimes a toddler's refusal to try a particular food is more about his need to experiment with control than with the actual taste of the food. It's often better to back off on the food and avoid the power struggle; at the next meal, substitute something equally nutritious.

Even with a one-year-old, you can begin to establish ground rules (see pages 89–93). It's *now* that you start, before the 'terrible twos' set in, at which point everything can turn into a power struggle.

Remember my B.A.R.N. acronym:

- The 'B' represents the various undesirable behaviours that occur at this age, behaviours that will persist if you don't step in now.

- The 'A' – your attitude – is critical. You'll notice that in each of the statements above describing a parent's concern about their child's behaviour, the implication is that *the child* is in charge. Granted, we're entering terrible-two territory now, but you have to take charge.

- Remember to look at the mealtime routine – the 'R' – which offers us a way of approaching the problem by actually *doing* things differently. It's important to set up structure and boundaries, particularly before 18 months, when truly obstinate behaviour often starts.

Teething: An Appetite Buster *cont'd*

Duration: Teething happens in 3-day increments – the time leading up to it, the tooth actually breaking through, and the aftermath. The worst 3 days are when the tooth is actually cutting through the gum.

What to do: Numb the gums with a teething salve. Your baby needs to chomp down. He may or may not be willing to suck on a frozen teether, a cold bagel, or a frozen facecloth.

No Games! No Coaxing!

Some parents make mealtime into playtime, but, if you put food on a spoon and 'fly' it through the air, don't be surprised if your toddler later tries to propel his food *without* the spoon.

Children should never be coaxed into eating. They'll eat when they're hungry. And when food is laid out before them. But they won't eat because we trick them into it, and it might accidentally cause them to develop negative feelings about eating.

The trick at this stage is to maintain a healthy balance, allowing your child to experiment and knowing what is developmentally realistic to expect from her. For example, if your child baulks at wearing a bib, give her a sense that she has a say in the matter. Offer her two bibs and say, 'Which one would you like to wear?' On the other hand, don't give her too many choices. Instead of *asking*, 'Do you want to eat?', simply say, 'It's time to eat.' If she says no, you still sit her at the table. If she's hungry, she'll eat. However, if she then acts up in any way, you take her out of the high chair and away from the table. Give her two chances and then wait until the next scheduled mealtime, when she'll definitely be hungry.

To some extent, fidgeting at meals, refusing to get into the high chair, or wanting to stand up in it, is just part of toddler territory. I have noticed, though, that mums who engage in contact and conversation with their children have less trouble in this arena. Try asking your child,

'Where are the potatoes?' or point out, 'The peas are green.' When she stops eating, or the moment she looks like she's about to stand up, immediately take her out of the high chair and say, 'Okay, lunch is over. Time to wash our hands.'

When a toddler is exceptionally wiggly or seems uncomfortable in his high chair, I suspect that the parents might be asking too much. **Do you put him in the high chair and make him wait until you prepare dinner?** Even five minutes is an eternity for an active toddler. Prepare his meal and get everything ready *before* you put him in the high chair. **Do you leave him in the high chair past his eating time?** If you keep him in his high chair after he's stopped eating, the high chair might start to feel like jail to him. Then there's the child who refuses to get into his high chair in the first place. Instead of getting exasperated or angry, try to figure out *why* he hates his high chair so much and then gently reintroduce him to it. **How old was he when you first put him in?** *Had he been sitting up on his own by then?* If you put a child into a high chair before he's able to sit up on his own for at least 20 minutes, he might get uncomfortable, fatigued and have a negative association with the high chair.

It's important to acknowledge a child's reluctance or fears. If your child kicks his feet, arches his back or squirms to get out the moment you put him in, take him out immediately. Say, 'I can see you are not ready to eat just yet.' Then try again in 15 minutes. Sometimes the problem is that parents don't give young children transition rituals – it's not respectful to whisk a child away from an activity and simply plop him into a high chair. He needs time to get into eating mode: use words ('It's time for lunch! Are you hungry? Let's clean up these blocks and get our hands washed.') and give a few moments for the words to sink in; approach him respectfully and then put the blocks away and help him wash his hands. Before you actually put him in the high chair, say, 'Okay, now I'm going to put you in your high chair.'

But if your child has become almost phobic about the high chair, take a few steps back. Make mealtimes a pleasure again. Start by sitting her on your knee to feed her. Then graduate to a side-by-side situation, using a child-sized table or booster seat at the big table. You can try the high chair again after a few weeks, but if she still resists, you might have to stick with the booster seat. By a year to 18 months many children prefer a booster chair at the table with the rest of the family anyway.

Making a child part of the family dining experience often goes a long way in promoting not only more cooperative behaviour but also a toddler's willingness to eat on their own.

If your child seems reluctant to feed herself, **What is your attitude about her feeding herself? Are you rushed at mealtimes? Are you worried about the mess she makes?** It makes me sad to see two-year-olds who are capable of putting food on a fork but whose parents are too rushed or too anal to allow them. If you act impatient, constantly clean her up or wipe the high chair table off *while* she's eating, it won't take her long to realise that this is not fun.

It's also a matter of readiness. **What do you mean by 'feeding himself'?** You may have to adjust your expectations. Most one-year-olds are capable of feeding themselves with their hands, but not with a spoon. If your child hasn't started hand-feeding, leave finger foods on her tray and she'll eventually get the idea.

Using a spoon or fork is a much more complicated bit of business: having the manual dexterity to hold the spoon, slide it under the food, lift it without turning it over and, finally, get it into her mouth. Most babies can't even start to attempt those manoeuvres until around 14 months. Before that, you can give her a spoon to play with. Eventually, she'll put the spoon into her mouth. When you see that, start to fill the spoon for her – ideally, with sloppy oatmeal that sticks to the spoon. Most of it will end up in her hair (and yours!), but you have to give her time to experiment and to miss her mouth entirely. Somewhere between 14 and 18 months, she'll start getting the food into her mouth.

Of course, no matter how ready your child is, no matter how relaxed you are, all children, at some point in toddlerhood, decide to wear their cereal or their spaghetti as a hat. **Did you laugh the first time your baby did it?** I know that it was a moment in time, and he was absolutely adorable and irresistible. The problem is, your reaction delighted him even more than the act of putting the cereal on his head. So he does it again, except you get increasingly angry, and he gets increasingly confused.

Toddlers like to throw things – the mere act is empowering to a child. He doesn't know the difference between throwing his ball and hurling a hot dog at you. If he's under age one, you don't make a big deal out of it – it's not meant to get your attention – but be clear that you don't find throwing food acceptable.

And when he does put food on his head, try not to laugh. Just say, 'No, you can't put food on your head. We eat our food.' And then take it away. But expect that it might take several incidents to change the behaviour. If you don't act now, I assure you that in the next stage, from age two to three, you'll be dealing with even worse behaviour at the dinner table.

CHAPTER ELEVEN

Food Fads and Other Annoying Traits

Two to Three Years

By now your child can eat – and should be eating – just about everything that the grown-ups eat. He is able to eat at the table, in his high chair or booster seat, and you should be able to take him to restaurants as well. The biggest problems come at around two, when everything and anything can become a power struggle. A lot depends on his nature and how you've handled previous problems, but, fortunately, as your child approaches the third-year mark, things usually become easier.

Common concerns at this point are of two types: poor or weird eating habits and mealtime misbehaviour.

Poor or Weird Eating Habits

In this category, I often hear the following:

My child is not a good eater.
My child hardly eats anything.
My child only eats snacks.
My child is on a hunger strike.
My child insists on eating foods in a particular order.
My child eats the same foods over and over and over.
My child can have a meltdown if his peas touch his potatoes.

I always ask parents to clarify what they mean by 'a good eater'. Is that a child who eats a lot? A child who eats everything? **Is this something new or did he always eat like this?** Individual differences in temperament, household environment and attitudes about food all affect kids' eating patterns. Some toddlers eat less than others, just as some are more sensitive to strong tastes or don't like to experiment with new foods. Some children relish food more than others. And some just have more bad eating days than others.

By this age, you should have a pretty good idea about who your child is and what's normal for him. If he's always been a reluctant eater, or eats less than his peers, be realistic. It's also perfectly normal for a child not to eat as much as he did the day before – he'll probably make up for it the next day. As long as your doctor gives him a clean bill of health, leave him to work it out on his own. If you keep offering good food, making mealtimes pleasant and showing an interest in good food yourself, he'll more likely eat better.

If your child was a good eater in the past and isn't now, what else is going on? Has he just learned to climb? Is he ill? Teething? Under stress? Any of those factors can make a good eater become less interested in food.

Is eating a social experience for your child? As long as no one is harping on at him to eat, being at the family dinner table can be a good experience for a reluctant eater. And it's even better when he's given the opportunity to eat with his peers. Surprisingly, even a poor eater becomes more attentive to food when he sees another child eating.

Is he really not eating *anything*? Parents tend not to count liquid intake or snacks in between meals. Keep track for a day or two of everything that goes into your child's mouth, and you might be surprised. Maybe he's a snacker. If so, he's eating – just not what you give him at mealtimes. You can take steps to correct that (see box, pages 126–127).

Food Fads

Even toddlers who get a good start on solids can sometimes get into what I call 'food fads' at this stage. Some eat the same food over and over. Others are peculiar eaters. Young children are particularly prone to food fads, both in the behavioural sense and also in their selection of foods. That's why it is so important that we give children healthy foods; at least the one food your child is getting will be good for her. Remember, too, that once a child has eaten her fill of a particular food, she'll frequently resist eating that food again for a very long time.

Quirky behaviour around food causes parents even more stress than repetitive eating patterns: a child not eating anything broken, or one who doesn't like anything 'mixed up' like stews or casseroles, a third who will eat only the top of a slice of toast, not the bottom. Some children insist on eating their food in a particular order – for example, one little boy absolutely had to start every meal with a piece of banana. Or, they have strict rules about what's put before them, that foods can't touch or that they have to be on a certain kind of dish or bowl.

The variations are endless and unique. *Why* they happen is anyone's guess. The only thing I can tell you for sure is that most kids grow out of them . . . eventually. If you react too strongly or put too much energy into trying to 'fix' your child's eating, you risk making it worse.

Mealtime Misbehaviour

The other kind of issues I hear at this age are similar to these:

My child has atrocious manners – what's okay at this age?
My child can't sit still at the dinner table (the 'wiggly worm syndrome').
My child throws food when she doesn't want any more or doesn't like it.
My child has tantrums at mealtime – the slightest thing can set her off.
My child purposely makes a mess, like painting the table with spaghetti sauce.

Many of these behaviour problems are an extension of similar issues that crop up during the day, but parents notice them more at dinner, especially when other people witness the scene. **Is this behaviour new, or has it been going on for a while? If the latter, in what other situations does it happen? What usually prompts it?** More often than not, the behaviour is not new; it's the result of accidental parenting. So let's say your child is finger-painting the table with spaghetti sauce. If you say nothing to your child, you're telling her it's okay. But then a few weeks later you're at Grandma's house and she starts 'decorating' your mother-in-law's heirloom tablecloth. You have to *teach* her that spaghetti sauce is not for finger-painting. The first time, you should have said, 'Food is for eating. You don't play with it. When you're finished eating, you take your plate to the sink.'

Whatever your child is doing that's unacceptable, be direct and tell her it's wrong: 'No, we do not [describe what she's doing] at the dinner table.' If she doesn't stop, excuse her from the table. You can invite her back in five minutes and allow her to try again.

It's the same with throwing food. It's one thing to see a 14-month-old experimenting with motion and throwing; it's best to make light of it (see page 134). But with a two- or three-year-old who's doing it to get a rise out of you, you have to tell him what he did was wrong, and make him clean it up. Take the plate away, saying, 'No throwing food.' Get him out of the chair and try again in five minutes. Give him two chances, and then he doesn't get anything.

This might sound stern, but children of this age know how to manipulate their parents. If you don't, it can turn into a longer-term problem, and you have a thrower on your hands who hurls not only food but toys and other potentially harmful objects. Who is going to teach him to be respectful – and when?

Sometimes, misbehaviour is solved by parents simply paying closer attention to their child's cues. **Do you watch for signs that your child is full?** Parents sometimes try to get children to eat 'one more bite' even though the kid is whining, turning his head away, kicking his feet. They keep trying, and eventually they have a meltdown on their hands. Instead, they need to take their child away from the table immediately.

Parents can unwittingly lay the seeds of more serious eating issues later on, so be careful about the unintentional messages you might give your child about food. Pushing her to eat more than her fill doesn't give her an opportunity to control her own body, or to know when she's full. Many overweight adults recall that they were given a lot of treats and praised for cleaning their plate and they quickly began to associate eating with parental approval. If you have eating issues yourself, be sure to acknowledge them and get help so that you don't pass them on to your child.

A well-fed baby or toddler is one who plays well and sleeps well. We owe it to our kids to give them the fuel they need and, at the same time, to respect their individual differences, even their idiosyncracies.

Index

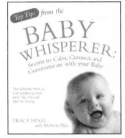
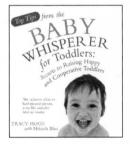

Also available from Vermilion

Tops Tips from the Baby Whisperer: Sleep

Handy tips from Tracy Hogg's practical sleep programme to help you overcome your baby's sleep problems.

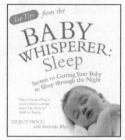

Price: £6.99

ISBN: 9780091929725

Top Tips from the Baby Whisperer: Potty Training

Essential advice on what you need to get started, getting your child into a routine and what to do if it doesn't go to plan.

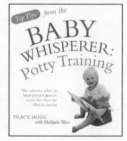

Price: £6.99

ISBN: 9780091929756

Order titles direct from www.rbooks.co.uk/babywhisperer